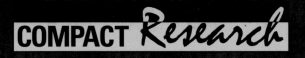
Meningitis

by Hal Marcovitz

Diseases and Disorders

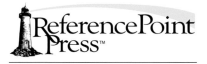

ReferencePoint Press™

San Diego, CA

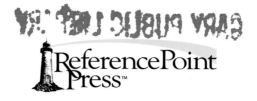

© 2009 ReferencePoint Press, Inc.

For more information, contact:
ReferencePoint Press, Inc.
PO Box 27779
San Diego, CA 92198
www.ReferencePointPress.com

Picture credits:
Maury Aaseng: 33–35, 49–52, 67–70, 86–89
AP Images: 11, 15

LIBRARY OF CONGRESS CATALOGING-IN-PUBLICATION DATA

Marcovitz, Hal.
  Meningitis / by Hal Marcovitz.
     p. cm. — (Compact research series)
  Includes bibliographical references and index.
  ISBN-13: 978-1-60152-043-2 (hardback)
  ISBN-10: 1-60152-043-3 (hardback)
  1. Meningitis—Popular works. I. Title.
  RC376.M37 2008
  616.8'2—dc22

                                                        2007045213

Contents

Foreword

66 **Where is the knowledge we have lost in information?** 99

—"The Rock," T.S. Eliot.

As modern civilization continues to evolve, its ability to create, store, distribute, and access information expands exponentially. The explosion of information from all media continues to increase at a phenomenal rate. By 2020 some experts predict the worldwide information base will double every 73 days. While access to diverse sources of information and perspectives is paramount to any democratic society, information alone cannot help people gain knowledge and understanding. Information must be organized and presented clearly and succinctly in order to be understood. The challenge in the digital age becomes not the creation of information, but how best to sort, organize, enhance, and present information.

ReferencePoint Press developed the *Compact Research* series with this challenge of the information age in mind. More than any other subject area today, researching current issues can yield vast, diverse, and unqualified information that can be intimidating and overwhelming for even the most advanced and motivated researcher. The *Compact Research* series offers a compact, relevant, intelligent, and conveniently organized collection of information covering a variety of current topics ranging from illegal immigration and methamphetamine to diseases such as anorexia and meningitis.

The series focuses on three types of information: objective single-author narratives, opinion-based primary source quotations, and facts and statistics. The clearly written objective narratives provide context and reliable background information. Primary source quotes are carefully selected and cited, exposing the reader to differing points of view. And facts and statistics sections aid the reader in evaluating perspectives. Presenting these key types of information creates a richer, more balanced learning experience.

For better understanding and convenience, the series enhances information by organizing it into narrower topics and adding design features that make it easy for a reader to identify desired content. For example, in *Compact Research: Illegal Immigration*, a chapter covering the economic impact of illegal immigration has an objective narrative explaining the various ways the economy is impacted, a balanced section of numerous primary source quotes on the topic, followed by facts and full-color illustrations to encourage evaluation of contrasting perspectives.

The ancient Roman philosopher Lucius Annaeus Seneca wrote, "It is quality rather than quantity that matters." More than just a collection of content, the *Compact Research* series is simply committed to creating, finding, organizing, and presenting the most relevant and appropriate amount of information on a current topic in a user-friendly style that invites, intrigues, and fosters understanding.

Meningitis at a Glance

Strains of the Disease

Meningitis can be spread through bacteria or viruses. The bacterial form is much more serious.

Transmission

Meningitis is contracted by coming into contact with the saliva or mucus from an infected person, usually through a cough, a sneeze, or a kiss, or by sharing a drinking glass, eating utensil, or cigarette.

Main Symptoms

High fever, nausea, vomiting, headaches, dizziness, stiff necks, and other joint pain are common among patients, but because the symptoms of meningitis often mimic the flu it could take a week before the results of a spinal tap provide definitive evidence.

Treatment

Bacterial meningitis patients receive large doses of penicillin or other antibiotics that are usually effective but the drugs are often unpleasant, carrying many side effects such as nausea, vomiting, diarrhea, skin rashes, fever, and difficulty breathing.

Severe Consequences

The U.S. death rate for meningitis is between 5 and 10 percent. The number is even higher in developing nations. Survivors may lose fingers, toes, hands, or legs. Long-term victims may suffer loss of hearing and eyesight, learning disabilities, dementia, and behavioral problems.

People Most at Risk

Babies and teenagers, particularly college freshmen living in dormitories, are most at risk for contracting meningitis; each year, about 125 college freshmen contract the disease.

Epidemics

Widespread epidemics are common in the so-called meningitis belt of sub-Saharan Africa; the last epidemic, which occurred in 1996, cost some 25,000 lives.

The Next Epidemic

Because of the cost and the logistical problems of delivering medicine over such a widespread area, international health care agencies may not be able to provide vaccinations to 50 million people in Africa during the next epidemic.

Vaccines

No meningitis vaccines are 100 percent effective, but one vaccine has virtually wiped out *hemophilus* meningitis in the United States and other industrialized countries.

Overview

Meningitis is an infection of the meninges, which are the thin membranes that surround the brain and spinal cord. When the meninges are infected they can become inflamed, leading to a number of symptoms. In most cases, people who get meningitis, also known as meningococcal disease, recover fully after a brief illness that is similar to the flu. In some cases, meningitis can lead to severe consequences, including loss of hearing, brain damage, loss of limbs, and death.

Indeed, meningitis can be a particularly deadly disease. According to the World Health Organization, the public health arm of the United Nations, meningitis afflicts some 500,000 people a year. That number is often larger in years in which epidemics sweep across Africa and other places that experience widespread outbreaks. Even in the United States, where vaccines and medical care are widely available, the disease afflicts some 1,200 people a year.

Meningitis can attack quickly and relentlessly. In many cases, meningitis is misdiagnosed as the flu. Victims feel ill for a day or two. When they drag themselves to the doctor or a clinic, they exhibit flu-like symptoms and are often advised to go home and go to bed. A day or two later, their conditions have grown worse but by then, it may be too late to save their lives.

A 2007 study by the University of Oxford in Great Britain found that half of all young victims of meningitis are sent home by their doctors who believe they are suffering from the flu. One British parent, Robert Leyland, had to fight to convince a doctor that his three-year-old daughter, Morgan, contracted something far more serious than the flu. "The doctor we saw just wouldn't listen," Leyland told the *London Telegraph*, "even when I held up a leaflet on meningitis that I'd found in the reception area and said Morgan had the symptoms listed."[1] Sadly, Morgan Leyland died of meningitis.

Bacterial and Viral

Meningitis can be spread by bacteria or viruses. A virus is an organism that is spread from one living thing to another. West Nile virus, for example, is spread through the bite of a mosquito. West Nile virus is one of several viruses that can cause meningitis.

Bacteria are organisms that can survive in a living thing or on their own—in the dirt or water or floating in the air. In most cases, bacteria are harmless but some bacteria can cause devastating diseases, such as tuberculosis, cholera, syphilis, and bubonic plague.

Viral meningitis is minor in most patients. Most patients recover in a week or 2. Bacterial meningitis is far more serious and can cause long-lasting effects. In about 8 percent of the cases, bacterial meningitis causes death within 48 hours. There are 4 known strains of bacterial meningitis—neonatal meningitis, hemophilus meningitis, meningococcal meningitis, and pneumococcal meningitis. At one time, hemophilus meningitis was the most prevalent form of meningitis, but an effective vaccine has been developed against the

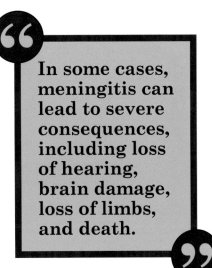

In some cases, meningitis can lead to severe consequences, including loss of hearing, brain damage, loss of limbs, and death.

disease. Still, hemophilus meningitis as well as the other strains of the disease remain a concern to public health officials.

Physicians diagnose meningitis by performing a spinal tap—they withdraw fluid from the spinal cord and examine it for infection. A person stricken with meningitis is treated with antibiotic drugs. Antibiotics have been used to treat bacterial infections following the discovery of penicillin in 1929 by Alexander Fleming, a Scottish biologist. Since then, other antibiotics have been developed but in recent years medical researchers have discovered that some bacteria have evolved and adapted to the drugs, making them ineffective. The bacteria that cause meningitis are among the germs that have adapted to antibiotic drugs, meaning that it is growing more difficult to fight the disease.

Dorm Disease

Most cases are spread by person to person contact through upper respiratory secretions, such as saliva or mucus from a runny nose. It can be spread through a cough, a sneeze, or a kiss, or by sharing a drinking glass, eating utensil, or cigarette. Meningitis is common in places where people live in close contact, such as college dormitories. A report by the U.S. Centers for Disease Control and Prevention (CDC), the federal agency charged with studying trends in public health, found that college students living in dormitories are 23 times more likely to contract meningitis as students who live at home, or in apartments or similar places where the concentration of students is lower than in the typical dormitory. In fact, the CDC found that 44 percent of all meningitis cases among college students are contracted by freshmen, who are more likely than older students to live in dormitories.

The bacteria that cause meningitis are among the germs that have adapted to antibiotic drugs, meaning that it is growing more difficult to fight the disease.

But that doesn't mean incoming freshman should fear their first experiences away from home. Most colleges recognize the public health issues of dorm life and urge freshmen and other students to get plenty of rest and eat well—which helps build up their immunities. College health officials also urge students to maintain healthy habits and lifestyles, by covering their mouths and noses when they cough and sneeze, and by refraining from sharing cups or utensils with others. Most colleges also require incom-

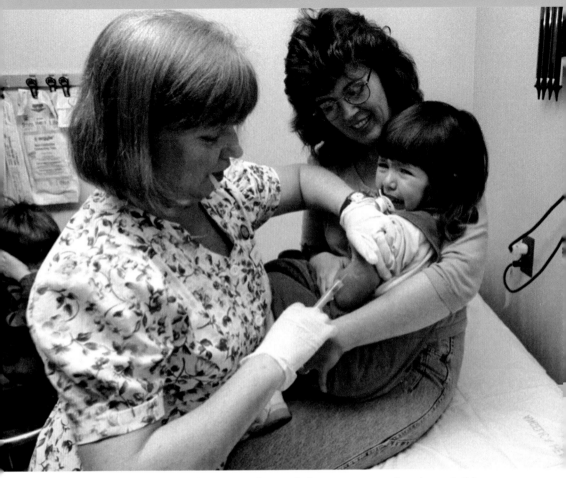

In 1998, Rhode Island parents demanded vaccinations for their children after 3 children died from meningitis within a 2-month span. In response to the demands, Rhode Island health officials made vaccinations available to some 274,000 children. This girl cries as she receives the vaccination.

ing students to obtain meningitis vaccines. Said Dr. Ralph Manchester, director of health services at the University of Rochester in New York, "College students need to be aware that this is a very serious disease that can strike without warning, and the only good strategy to decrease their risk is to get the vaccine before they get into the high-risk period in the first year, in a residence hall."[2]

Others at Risk

Newborn babies are also at high risk to contract meningitis. Their immune systems may be compromised by a number of factors, particularly low birth weight, which could have been a result of a premature birth or the poor health habits of the mother during pregnancy such as smoking, drug abuse, or poor diet. Newborns may also be susceptible to meningitis if they are born with damaged meninges, or if they come into contact with a nurse or other hospital worker who has contracted the disease but may not be showing symptoms. According to the CDC, of the 1,245 cases of meningitis reported to the agency in 2005, 151 cases—more than 10 percent—were contracted by victims less than one year old.

Viruses and bacteria are the primary causes of meningitis but not the only ones. For example, people who suffer traumatic head injuries are often susceptible to meningitis. Such incidents as accidental falls, car collisions, assaults, and gunshot wounds could rupture or cause inflammation to the meninges, which could lead to meningitis. Reported the *Internet Journal of Neurosurgery*, "Post-traumatic meningitis can lead to devastating results and mortality rates up to 65 percent have been reported. While the time between injury and infection may be brief, there are numerous cases where post-traumatic meningitis has been diagnosed years after the injury."[3]

Sub-Saharan Africa

In the United States and other industrialized nations, most people have access to health care that can help prevent the spread of meningitis or cure the disease before it becomes life threatening. That is not always the case in the developing world. People who live in impoverished countries, particularly in Africa, have endured widespread epidemics of meningitis.

> **Meningitis is common in places where people live in close contact, such as college dormitories.**

In fact, public health officials call a large portion of sub-Saharan Africa—the region of the continent below the Sahara Desert—the "meningitis belt" because there have been 3 significant epidemics of the disease since the 1970s. The last epidemic, which occurred in 1996, afflicted more than 250,000 people and caused some 25,000 deaths. Since then, meningitis has continued to afflict sub-Saharan Africa; from 1997 to 2002, another 223,000 Africans contracted the disease. What's more, the World Health Organization (WHO) believes the meningitis belt is expanding, reaching farther into the continent, and that a new epidemic may be approaching. Said a 2007 WHO report, "2006 . . . saw a significant increase in outbreaks of meningitis across the African meningitis belt. The increase in attack rates in countries where the incidence has remained low for several years, such as Mali, Nigeria and Sudan, is particularly worrying. The association of these epidemiological factors with the emergence of a new strain . . . in several countries in the belt makes it highly likely that a new epidemic wave will emerge in the coming years."[4]

> " The World Health Organization believes the meningitis belt is expanding, reaching farther into the continent [Africa], and that a new epidemic may be approaching. "

If a new epidemic occurs in Africa, the WHO believes it is prepared. From January to March in 2007, an outbreak of meningitis in the African nation of Burkina Faso afflicted more than 22,000 people, causing nearly 1,500 deaths. However, by early April, the crisis was brought under control after the WHO rushed nearly 3 million doses of meningitis vaccine to the country.

How Does Meningitis Affect People?

People who contract meningitis often believe they have the flu because the symptoms are similar. The victims may start out with fever followed by nausea, vomiting, headaches, and dizziness. Joint pain is common in meningitis, particularly in the neck. Meningitis sufferers are sensitive to light. They may also become disoriented.

College student Janet Cornebise described her symptoms to *Current Health 2* magazine: "I thought I was coming down with the flu. It was just before finals in my freshman year of college, so I was pretty stressed out. Then one night I got an unbelievable headache and my ears wouldn't stop ringing. I spent the night in the bathroom, throwing up and crying for my mom. The next morning my friends in the dorm took me to the clinic. When the doctor tried to push my head down to my chest, I screamed. They did a spinal tap, which I didn't even feel because my head hurt so much. I spent the next 10 days in the hospital with penicillin dripping into me."[5]

If the patient develops a form of meningococcal disease known as meningococcemia, the results can be far more serious. In meningococcemia, the disease is caused by the same bacteria that causes meningitis, but it does not infect the meninges. Instead, the disease spreads into the blood and infects other parts of the body. Doctors may notice red spots on the abdomen, which are caused by blood leaking out of the capillaries. The loss of blood could cause the liver and kidneys to shut down, which could cause death. Other parts of the body are affected by the loss of blood. If the patient recovers from the infection, the loss of blood may cause tissue to die. It is not unusual for meningococcemia victims to lose fingers or toes or even arms and legs. A form of brain damage known as dementia may also occur. Dementia patients have decreased powers of memory. Hearing and eyesight loss is also common among meningococcemia victims.

Death Rate

The loss of blood to vital organs is one way in which death may result from meningitis. The disease has other ways of killing its victims. They may slip into a deep coma from which they cannot be revived. Or they may suffer from septic shock, which is when blood pressure drops to a dangerously low level. Meningitis may cause respiratory failure, meaning the person cannot draw enough breaths to stay alive. Meningitis can also cause seizures of the brain, which are sudden bursts of activity that often cause the whole body to suffer shocks or jolts. Repeated brain seizures can cause unconsciousness and death.

> It is not unusual for meningococcemia victims to lose fingers or toes or even arms and legs.

Typically, the most severe forms of bacterial meningitis cause death in 5 to 10 percent of cases. The mortality rate is higher in the meningitis belt and other developing countries, where death may result in 20 percent of people with the disease. Dr. James Turner, director of student health for the University of Virginia, told the PBS documentary series *Nova*, "It's

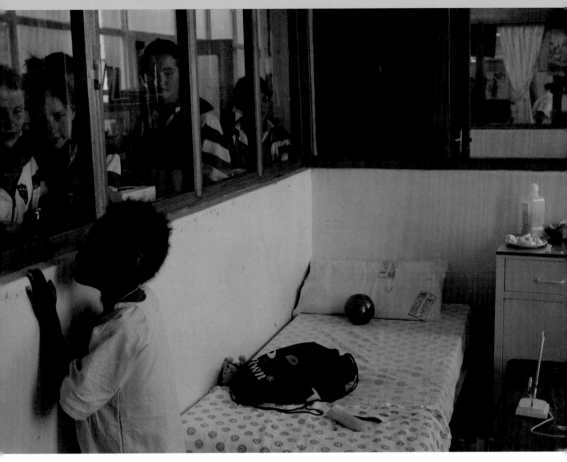

Meningitis is an infection of the meninges, which are the thin membranes that surround the brain and spinal cord. When the meninges are infected they can become inflamed, leading to a number of symptoms. This infected child is in isolation in a hospital in Johannesburg, South Africa.

the only infectious disease that I'm aware of that can take an otherwise healthy individual, and within four or five hours they're hospitalized, in an intensive care unit, in shock, on a ventilator, clinging to life."[6]

What Are the Social Impacts of Meningitis?

Meningitis can have a devastating effect not only on the person who is ill but also on that person's family, friends, and local community. Minimally, a college education may have to be interrupted because it could take weeks or even months for the patient to regain health. In the meantime, he or she may have to drop out of school and stay home, where parents may be forced to miss work to care for their son or daughter.

If the disease leaves a debilitating impact on the body, the effects could last a lifetime. A promising young person facing a bright future suddenly finds himself or herself handicapped by the disease. One outcome could be hearing loss, which would require special education classes. Young athletes may be confined to wheelchairs after losing limbs. A home may have to be remodeled so that the entrances, bathrooms, and other facilities are made wheelchair-accessible. Sometimes the medical costs could bankrupt a family.

Whether the effects of the disease wear off after a few months or remain for a lifetime, victims may often find themselves cut off from their friends, the activities they enjoy doing, and the places they enjoy visiting. The disease has a way of leaving patients lonely and feeling depressed.

Effect on Children

Young children who survive a bout of meningitis may continue to face ill effects as they grow older. A study performed in 2001 by a group of British physicians assessed the long-term impacts of meningitis on some 1,400 people who contracted the disease in the late 1980s and survived past the age of 5. They found a large percentage of the survivors suffering from a number of ills, both mental and physical, including learning disabilities, seizure disorders, hearing problems, partial or complete blindness, speech impediments, and behavioral problems.

"The most common [behavioral] problems among children who had had meningitis were severe temper tantrums, hyperactivity, and having poor concentration or being slow at school," wrote the authors of the study, published in the medical journal *BMJ*. "Among the 32 children classed as having poor concentration or being slow at school there was no other apparent health problems."[7]

The authors of the study revisited the study participants in 2007. By now, they had grown into young adults. This time, the researchers found symptoms of learning disabilities and other ills in more of the former meningitis patients than they had identified six years before. "It is alarming that children who appeared to have escaped meningitis unscathed when assessed at age 5 did no better in their [school] examinations than those with recognized disabilities,"[8] one of the study's authors, Dr. John de Louvois, told the Reuters news service.

Communities May Panic

Since meningitis may cause such devastating consequences, many communities often find themselves in the midst of a panic when even a single case occurs. Indeed, in fall 2007 a student at Appalachian State University in North Carolina came down with the flu. A rumor quickly spread throughout the student's dormitory that she had contracted meningitis, and within hours students were lined up at the university's health center, requesting vaccinations. It turned out that the student did not have meningitis—she really did have the flu. One of the dorm residents, Kimberly D. Canady, told a reporter for the student newspaper that when she heard the rumors of the meningitis case she realized she had not been vaccinated before enrolling. "The first thing that went through my mind was not having the vaccination," she said.[9]

> Since meningitis may cause such devastating consequences, many communities often find themselves in the midst of a panic when even a single case occurs.

Of course, officials at the university health center were only too happy to administer the vaccine, pointing out that all students should obtain the immunizations before starting classes.

If the mere rumor of a meningitis case can cause long lines to form at a health clinic, news of an actual outbreak can cause even more concern. When the media report a death caused by meningitis, local health authorities often find themselves inundated with phone calls from concerned people. In 1998, Rhode Island parents demanded vaccinations for their children after 3 young people died from the disease within a 2-month span. In response to the demands, Rhode Island health officials made vaccinations available to some 274,000 children. A year later, an outbreak of meningitis prompted parents in Wales to march in the streets, demanding the government make vaccinations available. Government leaders responded by organizing a mass vaccination program throughout many Welsh communities.

Can Meningitis Be Prevented?

Public health officials and doctors advise people, particularly students, to take precautions. They suggest that practicing good health habits, such as not sharing cups or eating utensils, is a good first step in preventing the spread of meningitis. Knowing how to recognize the symptoms is also important.

> If the symptoms are recognized in time and treated with the appropriate antibacterial drugs, there is no reason a meningitis patient can't expect a full recovery.

But vaccinations are still the best method of preventing the spread of meningitis. The most widely used vaccine for meningitis is believed to be 85 to 90 percent effective in preventing infection. That vaccine is particularly effective against hemophilus meningitis. Since its introduction in 1990, the vaccine has greatly reduced the spread of the disease. Three other vaccines have fallen short of 100 percent effectiveness; nevertheless, physicians still urge young people and others who may be susceptible to the disease to seek immunizations.

There is no question that meningitis is a dangerous disease that can strike quickly, causing severe and unpleasant symptoms and even long-term consequences. And, certainly, death is always a concern when meningitis is diagnosed in a patient. Still, if the symptoms are recognized in time and treated with the appropriate antibacterial drugs, there is no reason a meningitis patient can't expect a full recovery. Said Dr. Phillip Barkley, director of student health services at the University of Florida, "Meningococcal disease and influenza, and other viral illnesses, share many of the same symptoms, including headache, fever, nausea and vomiting, and rash. Often, though, meningococcal disease will come on very suddenly and progress very rapidly. That's why it's incredibly important if students, their family, or friends recognize and see these symptoms, particularly if they're coming on quickly, to make sure they get medical help immediately." [10]

How Does Meningitis Affect People?

❝I remained sedated for a week and a half, and after spending a total of two months in the hospital, I recovered. My circulation was so bad, I needed six surgeries to remove dead tissue and had three fingers on my right hand amputated, which meant I had to relearn how to write. I suffered nerve damage, and my muscles atrophied from spending so much time in bed, so I had to relearn how to walk.❞

—Timber Eaton, a 22-year-old student at Oklahoma State University who contracted meningococcemia.

College freshman Maggie Lutz entered her first year at the University of Iowa with some worries about leaving home for the first time. Soon, though, she found herself enjoying her new-found independence and freedom. "I was going to lots of parties and having a blast,"[11] she told *Cosmopolitan* magazine. She also neglected her studies, so at the end of the second semester, as finals approached, Lutz was forced to spend hours cramming for tests.

One morning, she woke up with a sore throat. Lutz thought she had caught a cold, but after a week the soreness persisted. Then, she started running a fever. By the time she dragged herself to the doctor a few days later, she had grown extremely weak, felt soreness in her joints, and suffered from nausea, vomiting, and diarrhea. She was so sick her two roommates had to help her out of bed.

"Then I noticed what appeared to be purplish black freckles on my legs," she told *Cosmopolitan*. "It looked like they were splattered with chocolate sauce. I licked my finger and tried to wipe off one of the freckles, but it didn't work. I thought, 'Ooh. That's not chocolate.' My body was sending out all these alarms, but I was so out of it (I would eventually learn that my blood pressure was very low and I was technically delirious) that I didn't feel any panic. I figured that I just needed some medicine to make these strange symptoms stop, so I started to get ready to go to the health center. Later, I was told that if I had stayed put, I probably would have died right there in my dorm room."[12]

> " By the time she dragged herself to the doctor a few days later, she had grown extremely weak, felt soreness in her joints, and suffered from nausea, vomiting, and diarrhea. She was so sick her two roommates had to help her out of bed. "

Lutz did not realize it at the time, but the moment she felt a scratchy throat, her life was about to take a dramatic turn. Lutz contracted bacterial meningitis. After arriving at the university's health center, she was quickly diagnosed with the disease and rushed to a hospital emergency room, where antibiotics were administered. She spent five weeks in the hospital, followed by a year at home to fully recover from the disease. Eventually, Lutz did return to college and graduate.

Different Strains

Lutz contracted meningococcemia, which is an infection of the blood. It is one of the most devastating forms of meningitis because the disease infects other parts of the body through the bloodstream and could damage vital organs. These organs, such as the kidney and liver, may shut down when they are denied blood, which may lead to the death of the patient. Meningococcemia victims who survive the disease often lose fingers, toes, or limbs because blood has been cut off from their extremities. It is a truly horrific disease.

The other forms of meningococcal disease can be just as devastating. Even the milder forms of the disease are far from pleasant. Other forms of meningococcal disease include hemophilus meningitis, meningococcal meningitis, neonatal meningitis, and pneumococcal meningitis.

Hemophilus meningitis is caused by the bacteria known as *Haemophilus influenzae* type b, or Hib. At one time, hemophilus meningitis was the most common form of the disease, but an effective Hib vaccine went into widespread use in 1990 and now the disease is much less prevalent. Even so, the vaccine is believed to be between 85 and 90 percent effective, which means some people who are inoculated still contract hemophilus meningitis. Of course, in places where vaccines are not readily available, such as the African meningitis belt, hemophilus meningitis is still a concern. Prior to the development of the vaccine, hemophilus meningitis was the most common form of meningitis found in young children and infants.

Meningococcal meningitis is more common in older children, teenagers, and young adults. It is caused by the bacteria known as *Neisseria meningitidis,* or *N. meningitidis.* Meningococcal meningitis has a high death rate—about 13 percent of victims succumb to the disease; nevertheless, all others usually recover with few long-lasting effects. *N. meningitidis* is also the bacteria that causes meningococcemia.

> " **Neonatal meningitis mainly afflicts newborn babies. It can be particularly devastating, killing as many as 50 percent of its victims if the disease is contracted within the first week of life.** "

Neonatal meningitis mainly afflicts newborn babies. It can be particularly devastating, killing as many as 50 percent of its victims if the disease is contracted within the first week of life. Infants contract the disease from their mothers or hospital workers. Premature babies or infants born with low birth weights are highly susceptible because their immune systems are not fully developed. The disease is caused by the bacteria known as Streptococcus group B and *Escherichia coli.*

Pneumococcal meningitis is not as prevalent as the other forms of the disease, but it is one of the most severe, causing death in some 30 percent of its victims. Caused by the bacteria Streptococcus pneumonia, the disease can be contracted by victims of all ages. It often enters the body through a respiratory infection or head injury.

How Is Meningitis Spread?

The bacteria that cause meningitis live in the back of the throat and in the nose. As such, meningitis is spread through a cough, sneeze, or kiss. People who share cups, eating utensils, or cigarettes can also spread the disease. Many people with strong immune systems can contract meningitis and never know they have it. Even if they haven't developed symptoms, they can still spread the germ by coughing in the direction of someone else, who breathes in the tiny specks of mucus floating in the air.

The bacteria that cause meningitis do not live long outside the body. That means it is unlikely meningitis can be contracted by swimming in the same pool as someone who has the disease.

Viral meningitis, which is usually a less severe form of the disease, is passed from one living thing to another. For example, West Nile virus, which can be contracted from the bite of a mosquito, can cause meningitis. There are many other viruses that can cause meningitis; indeed, the same virus that can cause the mumps or herpes can also cause meningitis. Victims of viral hepatitis usually recover after an illness of one or two weeks.

How Does Meningitis Attack the Body?

The brain is one of the most vital organs of the human body. It controls thought, intelligence, speech, breathing, movement, and virtually all other functions of the body. It is also one of the most fragile organs in the body. A brain injury can have a devastating effect on a person, leaving him or her comatose, unable to communicate, or impaired in any number of ways.

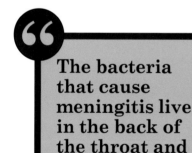

The bacteria that cause meningitis live in the back of the throat and in the nose.

The spinal cord is a bundle of nerves that carry the brain's commands to the rest of the body. It begins at the base of the brain and runs down a person's back, enclosed in the bones of the spine. The spinal cord is also a very fragile part of the body.

As such, nature has provided protection for the brain and spinal cord by enclosing them in the meninges, which are actually three wafer-thin membranes. The outer layer, which is tough and leathery, is known as the dura mater. The inner membrane is the arachnoid mater; it is an elastic layer lined on both sides by fluid known as cerebrospinal fluid, or CSF. Finally, the innermost membrane is known as the pia mater. This layer rests against the surface of the brain, following its many bumps, folds, and wrinkles.

When bacteria and viruses enter the human body, they may attack any number of organs or other parts of the body. Before it was virtually wiped out by an effective vaccine, the polio virus attacked human nerves and muscles, often leaving its patients crippled. The viruses that cause hepatitis attack the liver, often causing the condition known as cirrhosis, which is a scarring. When the liver is scarred, it cannot receive an adequate

> **Doctors can diagnose meningitis by performing a spinal tap.**

supply of blood and could shut down, causing death. Tuberculosis is caused by bacteria that attack the lungs, making it difficult for patients to breathe. Before a vaccine was developed in the 1940s, tuberculosis claimed millions of victims. Of course, not all viruses and bacteria are deadly. When a cold virus enters the body, it may leave the sufferer with a runny nose and scratchy throat for a few days, then disappear.

What Are the Symptoms?

Meningitis occurs when the three layers surrounding the brain and spinal cord are attacked by viruses or bacteria, causing them to become inflamed. Doctors can diagnose meningitis by performing a spinal tap. To perform the procedure, a doctor will insert a long needle into the spinal column, piercing the dura mater, so that a sample of CSF can be withdrawn. In the hospital lab, the CSF can be analyzed for the bacteria or viruses that cause meningitis.

The spinal tap is performed because patients usually exhibit symptoms that closely resemble the flu. Fever, severe headache, vomiting, confusion, drowsiness, and stiff neck are all common symptoms. In some cases, meningitis causes brain seizures or sensitivity to bright lights. Usually, it takes between two and 10 days before symptoms appear. Paul A. Offit, an infectious disease expert at Children's Hospital in Philadelphia, told the *Philadelphia Inquirer*, "It can be hard to distinguish meningococcal disease from a flu, which is why when people die, it's usually because it's not recognized soon enough."[13]

One symptom of meningococcemia is the rash that Maggie Lutz described as splatters of chocolate sauce. The rash is caused by blood leaking out of capillaries. If a doctor sees the rash, he or she can perform what is known as the tumbler test. The doctor will take a glass tumbler and press it against the rash, then look through the bottom of the glass. If the rash fades under the pressure, it is not meningitis. If the rash remains, the doctor is likely to order a spinal tap—if one has not already been performed.

> **Meningitis is the fifth most common cause of death among diseases caused by bacteria or viruses, following AIDS, tuberculosis, and two forms of hepatitis.**

Can Meningitis Be Fatal?

Anne Ryan, 19, was an otherwise healthy student at the University of Pennsylvania in Philadelphia. She wasn't even living in a dormitory— a sophomore, Ryan had moved out of the dorms for her second year at school, sharing an off-campus apartment with friends.

But soon after classes commenced in fall 2007, Ryan started feeling ill. Finally, on a Saturday afternoon, she checked herself into the Hospital of the University of Pennsylvania. She was soon diagnosed with meningococcal meningitis and died the next morning. Meningitis causes about 160 deaths a year, according to the U.S. Centers for Disease Control and Prevention. Meningitis is the fifth most common cause of death among diseases caused by bacteria or viruses, following AIDS, tuberculosis, and two forms of hepatitis.

In Ryan's case, university health officials as well as public health officials in Philadelphia and the student's hometown of Erie, Pennsylvania, made efforts to find anybody who may have been in contact with her during the final two weeks of her life. They were concerned that Ryan may have contracted the disease from a friend, who may have been passing the bacteria to others. After a brief investigation, though, health officials were unable to turn up anybody else exhibiting symptoms of meningitis. "We'll probably never be clear how she got it,"[14] Charlotte Berringer, director of community health for the Erie County Health Department, told the *Philadelphia Inquirer.*

Ryan may also have been a victim of a misdiagnosis, which is common in meningitis cases. Many physicians are also fooled by the symptoms, believing the patients are simply suffering from bad cases of the flu. In Ryan's case, an emergency room doctor sent Ryan home from the hospital, believing she had nothing more than a nasty case of the flu. Two days later, Ryan returned to the emergency room—this time much sicker. She was admitted—and died the next morning. Later, Ryan's family hired an attorney to determine whether she received adequate care in the emergency room. The attorney, Thomas Kline, told the *Philadelphia Inquirer*, "The one thing I can tell you without equivocation is the diagnosis was wrong."[15]

Other Causes of Meningitis

The meninges can become inflamed by causes other than infections. People who suffer head trauma through accidents, criminal acts, or other mishaps may develop the symptoms of meningitis because their meninges have become damaged and inflamed. Certain types of cancer attack the meninges, and this condition can lead to meningitis. Some people who take over-the-counter painkillers such as ibuprofen or naproxen may develop adverse reactions to the drugs that include inflammation of the meninges.

In addition, the disease known as listeria can develop into meningitis. The disease is caused by the bacteria known as listeria monocytogenes, commonly found in soil, dust, and food—particularly soft cheeses, hot dogs, and cold cuts. Also, many animals carry the bacteria, which means that people who work around animals, such as farmhands, are susceptible.

> " Some people who take over-the-counter painkillers such as ibuprofen or naproxen may develop adverse reactions to the drugs that include inflammation of the meninges. "

Listeria can have devastating consequences for pregnant women because the disease can infect their fetuses, resulting in the babies dying at birth or shortly after they are born.

Meningitis can develop into other diseases, particularly encephalitis, a swelling of the brain. Patients who suffer from encephalitis may become feverish, nauseous, confused, and sleepy. They may have difficulty walking or forming words or suffer from intense nightmares. There are few drugs that are effective in treating encephalitis. Instead, doctors usually treat the symptoms, such as providing painkillers for the headache and anti-inflammatory drugs to help reduce the brain swelling. Although severe cases of encephalitis can result in respiratory failure, coma, and death, most victims are able to recover from the disease in a few weeks.

As the cases of Timber Eaton, Maggie Lutz, and Anne Ryan prove, meningococcal disease can have devastating consequences—even for its survivors. The disease strikes quickly, relentlessly, and without warning. All three students knew they were very sick and in need of medical attention. Sadly, for Ryan, her symptoms fooled her doctors—a common and unfortunate outcome of a truly horrific disease.

How Does Meningitis Affect People?

66 They had to do a spinal tap on me and study the bacteria in a Petri dish. They began sticking me with so many needles that I felt like a voodoo doll. 99

—Maggie Lutz, quoted in Hannah McCouch, "I Almost Died of Dorm Disease," *Cosmopolitan,* April 2002.

Lutz, a University of Iowa student, contracted meningococcemia near the end of her freshman year.

66 There are some patients where it's amazingly obvious that they have [meningitis], but those patients are a rarity. 99

—Dr. Nancy Messonnier, quoted in Rebecca Kaplan, "Student Death: Experts Say Health Case Unlikely to Go to Court," *Daily Pennsylvanian*, October 11, 2007.

Messonnier is chief of the meningitis branch of the U.S. Centers for Disease Control and Prevention.

* Editor's Note: While the definition of a primary source can be narrowly or broadly defined, for the purposes of Compact Research, a primary source consists of: 1) results of original research presented by an organization or researcher; 2) eyewitness accounts of events, personal experience, or work experience; 3) first-person editorials offering pundits' opinions; 4) government officials presenting political plans and/or policies; 5) representatives of organizations presenting testimony or policy.

66 This isn't a disease that is passed through casual contact, like shaking hands. It spreads through prolonged face-to-face contact, by sharing drinking glasses or eating utensils—activities you find more often among children and in college dormitories. 99

—Charlotte Berringer, quoted in David Bruce, "Meningitis: Student Scourge Can Kill If Not Treated Promptly," *Erie Times News*, September 10, 2007.

Berringer is director of community health at the Erie County, Pennsylvania, Department of Health.

66 About 125 college students are hit with meningococcal disease every year, and as a result many of them will die, and even those who survive are often left with long-term health problems. 99

—Dr. Ralph Manchester, quoted in American College Health Association, "Meningitis on Campus." www.acha.org.

Manchester is director of health services for the University of Rochester in New York.

66 Living in crowded living conditions, such as dormitories, learning in crowded lecture halls, and lifestyle issues, such as kissing, smoking, sharing cigarettes, and patronizing bars, places [students] at increased risk. 99

—Dr. James Turner, quoted in American College Health Association, "Meningitis on Campus." www.acha.org.

Turner is director of student health for the University of Virginia.

❝Newborns and young infants may not have the classic signs and symptoms of headache and stiff neck. Instead, they may cry constantly, seem unusually sleepy or irritable, and eat poorly.❞

—Mayo Clinic, "Meningitis." www.mayoclinic.com.

The Mayo Clinic in Rochester, Minnesota, is one of the nation's premier medical treatment and research centers.

❝There's nothing more intense than the 24 hours when a patient comes in with meningococcal [disease]—the battle between life and death. They literally hang on to the edge of a cliff just waiting to fall over.❞

—Dr. Brett Giroir, quoted in *Nova*, "Killer Disease on Campus," 2002. www.pbs.org.

Giroir is a physician and medical researcher at Children's Medical Center of Dallas, Texas.

❝The rash is a little bruise caused by the blood leaking out of these small blood vessels in the skin that are being damaged by the disease process. But it's happening throughout the whole body, in every organ and every tissue base in the body.❞

—Dr. Ivan Dillon, quoted in *Nova*, "Killer Disease on Campus," 2002. www.pbs.org.

Dillon is a physician and medical researcher at St. Mary's Hospital in London, England.

66 Ninety-three percent of all children with meningococcal disease have the rash. And sometimes if the rash is severe it can compromise blood supply to the hands and feet. 99

—Dr. Joseph Britto, quoted in *Nova*, "Killer Disease on Campus," 2002. www.pbs.org.

Britto is a pediatrician who practices in London, England.

66 Obviously, one of the questions that gets a lot of interest from the teenagers is when you ask them how many people they've kissed. But kissing is thought possibly to be one way in which the bacteria can be transmitted among groups. 99

—Dr. Martin Maiden, quoted in *Nova*, "Killer Disease on Campus," 2002. www.pbs.org.

Maiden is a staff member of the Wellcome Trust Centre, a medical research organization, in Oxford, England.

66 The microbe colonizes only Man . . . and lives harmlessly in the main at the back of the human throat. Yet when it invades, it can cause disease of almost unparalleled ferocity, manifesting mainly as meningitis. 99

—Keith Cartwright, foreword to Matthias Frosch and Martin C.J. Maiden, eds., *Handbook of Meningococcal Disease*. Weinheim, Germany: Wiley-VCH, 2006.

Cartwright is an author who has written extensively on meningitis.

66 Raleigh carried me to the car, and he and Becca rushed me to a Stillwater hospital. By the time I got there, I couldn't move my neck—my head was hanging there like it was broken—a symptom of meningitis.**99**

—Sam Ellerbach, quoted in Beth Shapouri, "I Almost Died in My Dorm Room," *Cosmo Girl*, October 2007.

Oklahoma State University student Sam Ellerbach contracted meningitis in 2007.

Facts and Illustrations

How Does Meningitis Affect People?

- Of the patients who recover from meningococcal disease, between **11 and 19 percent** suffer permanent hearing loss, loss of limbs, brain damage, or other long-term effects, according to a 2005 report by the U.S. Centers for Disease Control and Prevention.

- A 2003 study by the World Health Organization found that between **10 and 25 percent** of the world's population is infected with the *N. meningitidis* germ, although most carriers of the germ do not get sick.

- Males and females are equally susceptible to meningococcal disease, according to the CDC. In 2005, the CDC reported, **618 males and 620 females** contracted meningitis.

- In 2002, Great Britain's Health Protection Agency reported that England and Wales suffer the highest rates of meningococcal disease in Europe, with nearly **2,800 cases a year**.

- Patients who are **65 or older** often contract pneumococcal meningitis. In many cases, the first symptom noticed by these patients is a severe earache.

- According to the American College Health Association, **between 5 and 15** college students die from meningitis each year.

- In 2007, the U.S. Food and Drug Administration approved use of a genetic analysis of spinal fluid that can provide evidence of viral meningitis within **three hours of the test**; previous tests took as long as a week.

- **Five percent** of cancer patients develop a secondary cancer in their meninges known as carcinomatous meningitis, according to Cancer Research UK, a British foundation that supports cancer research. Carcinomatous meningitis is most common in breast cancer patients.

- According to the National Foundation for Infectious Diseases, about **15 percent** of meningitis patients also develop pneumonia; most patients who develop secondary infections are older adults.

The Brain and Spinal Cord

The brain controls thought, intelligence, speech, breathing, movement, and many other functions of the human body. Its signals are transmitted to the parts of the body by the spinal cord, which is a bundle of nerves that runs down the back. Meningitis does not directly attack the brain and spinal cord, but the meninges—the layers that surround them. Even so, when the body is infected by meningitis a patient can suffer symptoms in the brain and spinal cord, including brain seizures, confusion, and a stiff neck.

Brain

Spinal cord

Source: Carolyn Gard, "What Is Meningitis?" *Current Health 2*, April/May 2003.

- Meningococcemia, the most serious form of meningococcal disease, has a fatality rate as high as **53 percent**, the National Foundation for Infectious Diseases reported in 2005.

- A University of Amsterdam study published in the *New England Journal of Medicine* in 2004 reported that **95 percent** of all meningitis patients suffer at least two of these symptoms: severe headache, fever, stiff neck, and altered mental status.

- Spinal taps are not foolproof: The University of Amsterdam study found that as many as **30 percent** of spinal taps in bacterial meningitis cases fail to indicate the infection in cerebrospinal fluid.

How the Brain and Spinal Cord Are Protected by the Meninges

When the brain and spinal cord are damaged, severe complications could occur, such as paralysis, inability to speak, dementia, and other ill effects. The brain is protected by three layers including the pia mater, arachnoid, and dura mater, collectively named the meninges. When these layers are infected by the bacteria or viruses, the patient often develops meningitis, which is an inflammation of the meninges.

Skull
Dura mater
Arachnoid
Pia mater

Meninges' layers

Source: Mayo Clinic Foundation for Medical Education and Research, Mayo Clinic, Rochester, MN. www.mayoclinic.com.

U.S. Deaths from Diseases Spread by Viruses, Bacteria, or Fungi

Meningococcal disease is the fifth-leading cause of death in the United States among diseases spread by bacteria, viruses, or fungi; 161 people died from meningococcal disease in 2003. The main cause of death by bacteria or virus is Acquired Immunodeficiency Syndrome (AIDS), primarily a sexually-transmitted disease that caused nearly 14,000 deaths in 2003. Toxic-shock syndrome, a bacteria-caused illness that afflicts women through tampons as well as birth control sponges and diaphragms, caused the lowest number of deaths. More than 70 victims died from the disease in 2003.

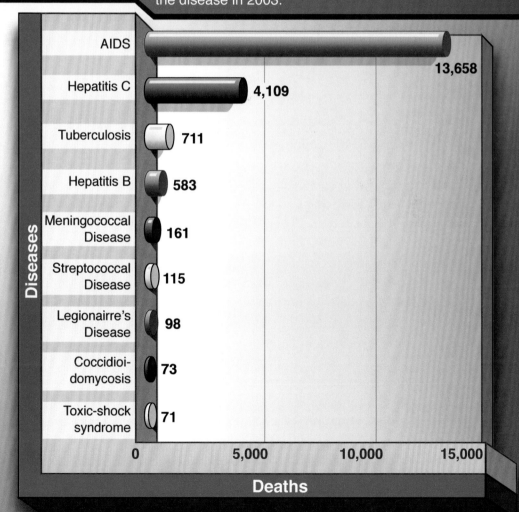

Diseases	Deaths
AIDS	13,658
Hepatitis C	4,109
Tuberculosis	711
Hepatitis B	583
Meningococcal Disease	161
Streptococcal Disease	115
Legionairre's Disease	98
Coccidioidomycosis	73
Toxic-shock syndrome	71

Source: U.S. Centers for Disease Control and Prevention, "Deaths from Selected Nationally Notifiable Diseases," *Morbidity and Mortality Weekly Report*, March 30, 2007.

How Prevalent Is Meningitis?

How Prevalent Is Meningitis?

66 In the dreary month of February, came the illness which closed my eyes and ears and plunged me into the unconsciousness of a newborn baby. 99

—Helen Keller, author and social activist.

Hippocrates, the Greek physician who lived in the fifth century B.C., first observed the symptoms of meningitis in his patients, meaning that the disease has existed in the human population for at least 2,500 years. Wrote Hippocrates, "If, during fever, the neck shalt have been sufficiently twisted, the [ability to swallow is] rendered difficult without any tumor, it is a fatal sign."[16] Hippocrates also correctly theorized that an injury to the lining of the brain could produce the symptoms.

Hippocrates and his successors understood little about germs and viruses and, therefore, never traced the disease to its true roots. In the centuries to follow, meningitis claimed many victims as physicians slowly started gaining an understanding of the disease and its horrific consequences. In 1661, British physician Thomas Willis determined that meningitis was the cause of an epidemic that was sweeping through England. He accurately described the symptoms and also suggested the disease may be linked to cerebrospinal fluid. In 1805, Swiss physician Gaspard Vieusseux reported the symptoms of a meningococcemia epidemic that struck Geneva, killing 33 people. He described common symptoms among the victims, including fever, vomiting, stiff neck, and skin rash. A year later, 2 Massachusetts physicians described the first known meningitis epidemic in America, which claimed 9 victims; and in 1807, Connecticut physician

Samuel Woodward published a description of the symptoms of meningococcemia in *The American Mercury*, a magazine of the era:

> The violent symptoms were great lassitude, with universal pains in the muscle; chills; heats, if any, were of short duration; unusual prostration of strength; delirium, with severe pain in the head, vomiting, with undescribable anxiety of stomach; eyes red and watery, and rolled-up, and the head drawn back with spasms; pulse quick, weak, and irregular . . . death often closed the scene in ten or fifteen hours after the first attack . . . the body near the fatal period, and soon after, became spotted.[17]

In 1887, Austrian physician Anton Weichselbaum made a breakthrough in the study of meningitis by linking it to infection by bacteria he cultured from a deceased patient's cerebrospinal fluid. Four years later, diagnosis of the disease took another step forward when German physician Heinrich Quinke perfected the spinal tap, enabling physicians to examine the CSF of living meningitis patients.

Noted Victims

Two of history's most noted victims of meningitis are Helen Keller and Oscar Wilde. Keller was born in 1880 to wealthy parents in Alabama. At the age of 19 months, she contracted a disease described as an "acute congestion of the stomach and brain."[18] The young girl's illness was regarded as grave; the family doctor predicted she would die but Keller survived the disease. "Early one morning," she wrote in her autobiography, "the fever left me as suddenly and mysteriously as it had come."[19] Still, the disease, which is believed to have been meningitis, left the young child blind and deaf.

> " In 1805, Swiss physician Gaspard Vieusseux reported the symptoms of a meningococcemia epidemic that struck Geneva, killing 33 people. "

Keller went on to lead a remarkable life, proving that handicapped people cannot be held back by their disabilities. She became an author and social activist, crusading for the rights of women, handicapped people, and others.

The young girl's emergence from the darkness of her disabilities was recounted in the Broadway play and Academy Award–winning film, *The Miracle Worker*, which told the story of Keller's relationship with her teacher, Anne Sullivan. Keller died in 1968, shortly before her eighty-seventh birthday.

> " Oscar Wilde lived a far shorter life, dying in 1900 at the age of 46. Meningitis robbed the English-speaking world of one of its most renowned writers. "

Oscar Wilde lived a far shorter life, dying in 1900 at the age of 46. The disease robbed the English-speaking world of one of its most renowned writers. Born in Dublin, Ireland, Wilde would go on to write the classic suspense novel *The Picture of Dorian Gray*, as well as the comedic play *The Importance of Being Earnest*. In October 1900, while living in France, he developed the symptoms of meningitis and died after an illness that lasted about 6 weeks. Ironically, the author's father, Sir William Wilde, was a physician who specialized in diseases of the ear, nose, and throat, and had studied meningitis, noting how symptoms of the disease affected the ear.

Epidemics Common

By the early years of the twentieth century, epidemics of meningitis were common. What's more, there was often little hope for the hapless patients who contracted the disease—few of them recovered. For example, a meningitis epidemic spread through Glasgow, Scotland, in 1907. Of 998 people who contracted the disease, 683 died. That same year, meningitis swept through Belfast, Northern Ireland, killing 493 people. Only 130 survived. Between 1899 and 1907, meningitis killed 90 percent of the young victims treated at Boston Children's Hospital. And during a meningitis epidemic in New York in 1904 and 1905, health authorities reported a staggering 5,000 deaths among the 6,700 cases of meningitis treated in the city.

The dramatic death rate would soon retreat. In 1908, the first of the so-called sulfa drugs was developed although the medications would not go into widespread use until the 1930s. These were the first antibiotic drugs. In 1935, a 10-year-old girl suffering from meningitis was treated with sulfa drugs at Columbia University Medical Center in New York; she was the first American to recover from the disease through the use of antibiotic medication. Still, the sulfa drugs were not quite miracle drugs; by the early 1940s, some 10 percent of meningitis patients still died from the disease. Indeed, between 1940 and 1945, meningitis took the lives of nearly 15,000 American servicemen, making it the leading cause of death for U.S. soldiers and sailors apart from combat.

The discovery of penicillin in 1929 by Alexander Fleming helped drive the death toll down as well, but meningitis still kills between 5 and 10 percent of its victims in the United States and other industrialized nations. In developing countries, particularly the African meningitis belt, the death rate is much higher—taking the lives of as many as 20 percent of the patients who contract the disease.

Still a Dangerous Disease

Indeed, throughout the world, meningitis remains a serious threat to public health, particularly in the African meningitis belt. Said a report by the World Health Organization, "The highest burden of meningococcal disease occurs in sub-Saharan Africa, which is known as the 'meningitis belt,' an area that stretches from Senegal in the west to Ethiopia in the east, with an estimated total population of 300 million people."[20] According to the WHO, the climate and weather conditions of the region help spread the bacteria, particularly the germ that causes the strain of the disease known as meningococcal meningitis. During the region's dry season, spanning from December through June, there is little rain and gusty winds, which helps spread airborne bacteria. What's more, the cold nights of the dry season often produce upper respiratory infections among the people who live there, which help break down their immunity and leave them vulnerable to other infections, such as meningitis.

> In 1935, a 10-year-old girl suffering from meningitis was treated with sulfa drugs at Columbia University Medical Center in New York; she was the first American to recover from the disease through the use of antibiotic medication.

The poverty of the region helps enhance the spread. Housing in many sub-Saharan countries is overcrowded, with many people living in close quarters. Food shopping is done in central, open-air marketplaces, where many people crowd around stalls. Said the WHO, "In major African epidemics, attack rates range from 100 to 800 per 100,000 population, but individual communities have reported rates as high as 1,000 per 100,000. While in endemic disease the highest attack rates are observed in young children, during epidemics, older children, teenagers and young adults are also affected."[21]

Nearly 4 out of every 100,000 babies born in the United States have contracted meningitis.

Who Is Most at Risk?

In industrialized countries, as in the African meningitis belt, anybody can contract meningitis but some people are more at risk than others. Because their immune systems are still developing, babies are regarded as highly susceptible to meningitis. According to the U.S. Centers for Disease Control and Prevention, nearly 4 out of every 100,000 babies born in the United States have contracted meningitis. As the children grow older and their natural systems of immunity develop, they are better able to fight off the infection without showing symptoms. The infection rate is lowest for children between the ages of 5 and 13—in that age group, just 1 child for every 200,000 is infected.

The rates start climbing again as young people enter their teen years. In the 14–24 age group, 1 person out of every 100,000 is likely to contract meningitis. That is the age group in which young people go away to college and where many of them live in dormitories, take classes in large lecture halls, and eat their meals in crowded college dining halls. In other words, they live and study in close contact with others. Darla Elder, director of student health services at Edinboro University in Erie, Pennsylvania, told the *Erie Times News*, "Students who live in the dorms are in close proximity to one another, and that is how the disease spreads."[22]

Party Lifestyle

But college students tend to place themselves at risk in other ways. Many young people who go away to college find themselves relishing their sudden independence from their parents. No longer are they told when they have to be home. Many of them stay out late at night—not just on weekends, but during the week as well. They may not get enough sleep and they may not eat nutritious diets, either. Perhaps they may let their studies go from time to time, then get little sleep as they cram before tests. Such habits are often acquired by freshmen, many of whom have not yet learned how to handle their new freedoms.

That sort of lifestyle helps break down their immune systems, making them more vulnerable to infections. Robin Kolble, a registered nurse and coordinator of the Student Wellness Program at the University of Colorado, told *Current Health 2* magazine, "As a mother, a nurse, and a health educator, I think that one reason freshmen in dorms are more at risk is because of poor life-management skills. They tend to have poor sleep habits, poor nutritional intake, and poor stress management skills."[23]

College is also an opportunity for students to attend many parties, where they may experiment with beer and other alcoholic beverages. They may also experiment with cigarette smoking as well as marijuana. Students may think little about sharing a beer or a glass of wine with a friend, or sharing their cigarettes with others. Smoking can also spread infection, because droplets of saliva may be exhaled in the smoke. Romantic relationships may blossom on a college campus as well. Therefore, college students are very prone to come into contact with the saliva or mucus of their friends or even complete strangers.

> " College is also an opportunity for students to attend many parties, where they may experiment with beer and other alcoholic beverages. . . . Therefore, college students are very prone to come into contact with the saliva or mucus of their friends or even complete strangers. "

Travelers Must Be Wary

People who travel to other countries where meningitis is common must be on their guard as well. Certainly, anybody traveling to countries in the African meningitis belt should be wary of conditions and take precautions, such as obtaining meningitis immunizations before departing.

But travelers from countries within the meningitis belt have been known to spread the disease. For example, each year some 2 million Muslim pilgrims make their way to the city of Mecca in Saudi Arabia to participate in the Hajj, a six-day religious ritual. The pilgrims pray together in close quarters; many of them live in a temporary tent city erected by the Saudi government on the outskirts of the city. Thousands of Muslim pilgrims leave their homes in the meningitis belt to attend the Hajj.

> Anybody traveling to countries in the African meningitis belt should be wary of conditions and take precautions, such as obtaining meningitis immunizations before departing.

Saudi Arabia has been hit by two recent epidemics of meningitis—in 1987 and 2000—and in both cases officials suspected the disease was introduced into the country by pilgrims participating in the Hajj. In the second outbreak, some 400 cases of meningitis were reported to Saudi public health authorities shortly after the Hajj. What's more, some pilgrims who returned to their homes in the United States, Great Britain, and elsewhere spread the disease as well. Liam Donaldson, chief medical officer for the British government, told BBC News, "Meningococcal infection is not only a serious threat to those traveling to the Hajj but also to their friends and family when they return."[24] Following the 2000 Hajj, the Saudi government started requiring pilgrims to obtain meningitis vaccinations before entering the country.

Meningitis has been a threat to human health at least since the era when Hippocrates first observed and noted the symptoms in one of his patients. Since then, the disease has afflicted many lives. Since Hippocrates' time, doctors have gained a greater understanding of the ailment and have found ways to treat the symptoms, but meningitis has proven to be one of the most resilient diseases known to mankind. It affects the health of students on college campuses in America, Muslim pilgrims making their annual treks to Mecca, and Africans who live in rural sub-Saharan villages. Despite many advances in medical science, meningitis has refused to go away.

Primary Source Quotes*

How Prevalent Is Meningitis?

❝Bacteria meningitis exacts a large physical, social, and economic toll on the world's children. This is especially true in developing countries, where greater rates of adverse outcomes are superimposed on poverty, other severe illnesses, and illiteracy.❞

—Dr. Keith Grimwood, "Legacy of Bacterial Meningitis in Infancy," *BMJ*, September 2001.

Grimwood is professor of pediatrics at the Wellington School of Medicine and Health Sciences in Wellington, New Zealand.

❝Drinking, smoking and not getting enough sleep all wreak havoc on the immune system.❞

—Dr. James C. Turner, quoted in Hannah McCouch, "I Almost Died of Dorm Disease," *Cosmopolitan*, April 2002.

Turner is director of student health for the University of Virginia.

---

* Editor's Note: While the definition of a primary source can be narrowly or broadly defined, for the purposes of Compact Research, a primary source consists of: 1) results of original research presented by an organization or researcher; 2) eyewitness accounts of events, personal experience, or work experience; 3) first-person editorials offering pundits' opinions; 4) government officials presenting political plans and/or policies; 5) representatives of organizations presenting testimony or policy.

Primary Source Quotes

❝I awoke after a tossing half sleep, and turned my eyes, so dry and hot, to the wall, away from the once-loved light, which came to me dim and yet more dim each day.❞

—Helen Keller, *The Story of My Life*. New York: Bantam Books, 1990.

Keller, an author and social activist, contracted meningitis at the age of 19 months, which left her blind and deaf.

❝Among children in developing countries, meningitis kills 20 percent of those infected, while up to 35 percent may go on to develop lifelong disabilities such as mental retardation or hearing loss.❞

—Dr. Adenike Grange, "Africa: Letter from Athens—Fighting for the World's Children," AllAfrica.com, August 24, 2007. http://allafrica.com.

Grange is minister of health for Nigeria.

❝People in the same household or day-care center, or anyone with direct contact with a patient's oral secretions [such as a boyfriend or girlfriend] would be considered at increased risk of acquiring the infection.❞

—U.S. Centers for Disease Control and Prevention, "Meningococcal Disease." www.cdc.gov.

The CDC is an agency of the U.S. government charged with monitoring threats to public health.

66 There is just something special about teenagers [and young adults]. They don't sleep right, they depress their immune system. They make conditions ideal for acquiring meningitis. 99

—Lynette Mazur quoted in Anissa Anderson Orr, "College Students and Meningitis," *University of Texas Health Science Center HealthLeader*, August 22, 2005. http://publicaffairs.uth.tmc.edu.

Mazur is professor of pediatrics at the University of Texas Medical School in Houston, Texas.

66 You see a story on the news about a case of meningitis at a nearby college, and it occurs to you that your favorite babysitter's brother goes there, and you wonder whether your child could have been exposed. 99

—Perri Klass, "To Worry or Not?" *Parenting*, November 2002.

Klass is a pediatrician and author.

66 Even if people are on medicine, they shouldn't have too much sense of security. This is a disease that can spread very quickly. 99

—Blaise Congeni, quoted in Debbie Howlett, "Meningitis, Terror Strike in Ohio: 2 Teens Are Dead from the Bacteria, and Residents Are Approaching Panic," *USA Today*, June 5, 2001.

Congeni is director of infectious diseases at Akron Children's Hospital in Akron, Ohio.

❝After several years of low disease incidence in the [meningitis] belt, the 2006 epidemic season saw a marked rise in meningitis attack rates across the region. This rise . . . across various countries are factors indicating that a new meningitis epidemic wave is beginning in Africa.❞

—*World Health Organization Weekly Epidemiological Record*, "Risk of Epidemic Meningitis in Africa: A Cause for Concern," March 9, 2007.

The World Health Organization is the public health arm of the United Nations.

....

❝It is particularly worrying that after 6–10 'silent' years, countries such as Mali, Nigeria and Sudan have experienced a significant increase in meningitis activity, which indicates that they might be simultaneously entering a new epidemic cycle.❞

—*World Health Organization Weekly Epidemiological Record*, "Risk of Epidemic Meningitis in Africa: A Cause for Concern," March 9, 2007.

The World Health Organization is the public health arm of the United Nations.

....

❝We found that adolescents and young adults accounted for a relatively high proportion of all cases of meningococcal meningitis and that infection in this age group led to death more often than expected.❞

—Dr. Lee H. Harrison, quoted in *Science Daily*, "Adolescents and Young Adults at High Risk for Deadly Meningitis, Says University of Pittsburgh–Led Study," August 8, 2001. www.sciencedaily.com.

Harrison led a University of Pittsburgh study that found young people between the ages of 15 and 24 accounted for 24 percent of meningitis cases among 295 studied as part of the test.

....

66 **Meningitis outbreaks take place after a period without rain, low humidity and lots of dust in the air.** 99

—Isabelle Jeanne, quoted in *Science Daily*, "Scientists Monitoring Dust Storms Linked to Health Risk," May 11, 2005. www.sciencedaily.com.

Jeanne, an epidemiologist for the Niger-based Center for Research Management and Environmental Studies, is part of a research team that uses satellite imagery to track dust storms in the meningitis belt, hoping to use the data to forecast the path of winds that carry bacteria.

Facts and Illustrations

How Prevalent Is Meningitis?

- According to Wayne Biddle's 2002 book *A Field Guide to Germs*, during World War I, the British army was so concerned about the spread of meningitis in the ranks that officials conducted studies to determine how much distance to place between bunks in the barracks to minimize infections among soldiers.

- Chinese New Year, which typically occurs in January or February, is a prime time for the spread of meningitis because many Chinese people travel to visit families, then contract the disease away from home. In January 2005, the BBC reported an outbreak of **258 cases in China**.

- Like students in America, young people in Europe are also susceptible to the spread of meningitis; a 2002 report by Great Britain's Health Protection Agency found that **13 percent** of all meningitis cases in Europe afflict people between the **ages of 15 and 19**.

- The World Health Organization has predicted a major meningitis epidemic may sweep through Africa sometime **between 2008 and 2010**, afflicting tens of thousands of victims, according to the Reuters news service.

- Four members of the Pittsgrove Township, New Jersey, High School football team **contracted viral meningitis** in fall 2007; it is believed they shared the same water bottle during a game or practice, according to the *Atlantic City Press*. A fifth student, who is not a member of the team, was also infected.

Affliction in Africa—the Meningitis Belt

The African meningitis belt stretches from Senegal in West Africa to Ethiopia in East Africa. Some 300 million people live in the belt, and they experience the highest rates of infection in the world. The poverty of the region is seen as a major reason for the high rate of infection—people endure crowded living conditions. Dry, dusty winds also spread bacteria in the air, adding to the danger.

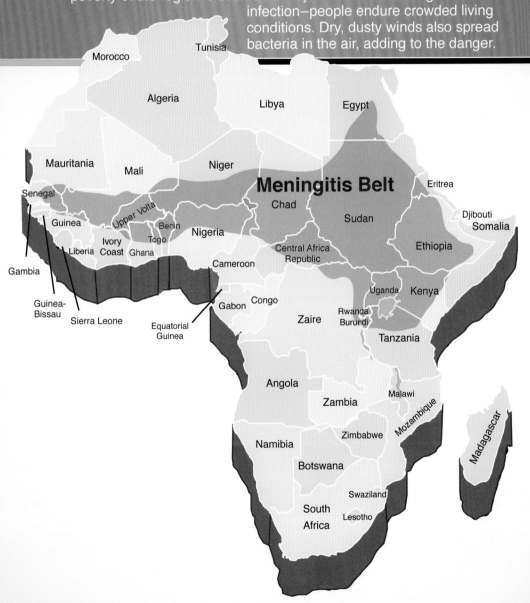

Source: Allan R. Tunkel, *Bacterial Meningitis*. Philadelphia: Lippincott, Williams & Wilkins, 2001.

- Despite Saudi Arabia's decision to bar Hajj pilgrims who have not been vaccinated against meningitis, many slip through. The *Lancet* reported the findings of a study that said **35 of 109 pilgrims** who traveled to Saudi Arabia from Great Britain in 2006 had not been vaccinated.

- **More than 80 people** in Massachusetts, New Hampshire, and Maine were advised to take antibiotics because they had come into close contact with 21-year-old college student Danielle Thompson shortly before she died from meningococcal disease in early 2007, the *New York Times* reported. Thompson had traveled extensively in those 3 states over winter break.

New African Epidemic Brewing

An epidemic in the African meningitis belt in 1996 and 1997 afflicted some 220,000 people. The World Health Organization rushed vaccines to the region, helping the infection rate to drop. New outbreaks in the meningitis belt in 2006 and 2007 have prompted WHO officials to predict that a new epidemic on the continent is brewing. In the first 3 months of 2007, some 22,000 new cases of meningitis were reported in the African nation of Burkina Faso, resulting in nearly 1,500 deaths.

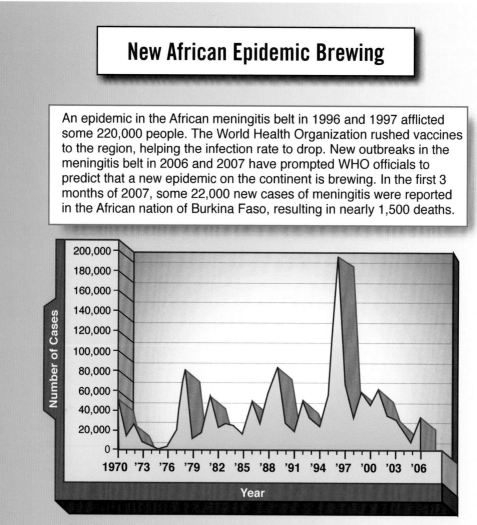

Source: *World Health Organization Weekly Epidemiological Record,*
"Risk of Epidemic Meningitis in Africa: A Cause for Concern," March 9, 2007.

U.S. College Freshmen in Dorms Most at Risk

About 33 percent of all college students who contract meningitis are freshmen who live in dormitories, according to a study performed in 1998 and 1999, and published in the *Journal of the American Medical Association* in 2001. That study showed 96 college students contracted the disease for the 12 months under the study, but since then the numbers have risen. According to the American College Health Association, in 2006 about 125 college students contracted meningitis.

Rates of Meningococcal Disease in College Students, 1998–1999

	Number of cases	Population	Rates per 100,000
All 18–23 year olds	304	22,070,535	1.4
College students	96	14,897,268	0.6
Undergraduate	93	12,771,228	0.7
Freshmen	44	2,285,001	1.9
Dormitory residents	48	2,085,618	2.3
Freshmen living in dormitories	30	591,587	5.1

Source: American College Health Association, 2001. www.acha.org.

- According to the U.S. National Center for Health Statistics, **about 1 in 200,000** Americans died from meningococcal disease in 2004.

- Viral meningitis is less severe than bacterial meningitis but it is still responsible for hospitalizing as many as **50,000 people** a year, according to the U.S. Centers for Disease Control and Prevention.

- Viral meningitis spread by mosquitoes was first discovered in the United States in 1999, when **59 cases** of meningitis and encephalitis caused by West Nile virus were diagnosed. The virus is spread by mosquitoes that bite infected birds and then bite humans.

Infection Rates Highest Among the Young

Babies are susceptible to meningitis because they have not developed strong immunities. As children grow older they are better able to fight off disease but once they reach their teen years, many start practicing risky behavior that compromises their natural immunity and makes them susceptible to infections, including meningitis. At age 14–24, meningitis infection rates begin to increase then drop off at the 25–64 age group.

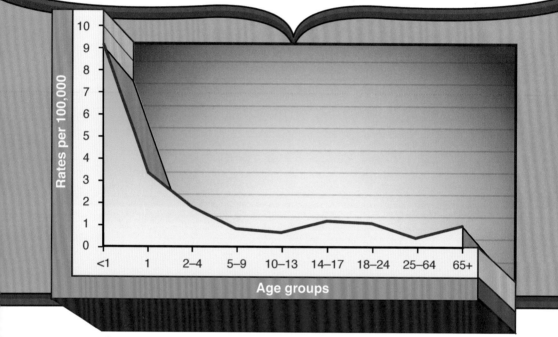

Source: American College Health Association. www.acha.org.

- Meningitis may be spread by **intimate contact**; in December 2004, seven gay men contracted meningitis in Vancouver, British Columbia.

- After one Rhode Island child contracted viral meningitis and three others contracted encephalitis, the state's Emergency Management Agency distributed **15,000 bottles of hand sanitizer** to Rhode Island schoolchildren to help ensure they would not spread germs, the *Providence Journal* reported in January 2007.

What Are the Social Impacts of Meningitis?

" Half the class is gone and half the school is not here— like, more than half. And, like yesterday, I wasn't allowed to come into school. I wasn't allowed this morning. I wake up, I got ready for school; my mom's like, 'You're not going.' I was like, 'I have to. I have exams.' **"**

—Dimitri Vasu, a student at Alliance High School in Alliance, Ohio.

College freshman John Kach had a bright future. He was on his way to becoming a star of the basketball team at Salve Regina University in Rhode Island. In the school's game against Bridgewater State University, Kach scored the winning basket. "Everything was, you know, going my way," Kach told the CBS News show *48 Hours*. "I was happy."[25]

Kach was a healthy and robust young man. He stood 6 foot 4 and weighed 210 pounds. That was before he started feeling ill from what he believed was the flu. "I was in my dorm room on a Friday night," he told *48 Hours*. "I wasn't feeling great, so I stayed in. All of a sudden, my stomach doesn't feel right . . . and then I started getting real hot, fever."[26]

In reality, the young student had contracted meningococcemia. As he battled the disease, the infection cut off the blood flow to his limbs. By the time he was released from a hospital six weeks later, doctors had been forced to amputate his right leg below the knee as well as his right hand.

Kach learned to live with his disabilities. He adapted to his prosthetic limbs but he will never play competitive college basketball again. His life was forever changed by meningococcal disease. His friends and family have also had to adapt as they help him learn to eat and walk again—activities he once took for granted.

Indeed, meningitis can have a devastating, lifelong impact on the victim as well as many others. Kach's mother, Paige Kach, told *48 Hours*, "Any parent sitting anywhere can't even imagine how horrible it is to have somebody say, 'We're going to cut off his hands, we're going to cut off his legs.' You're a beautiful child. You're a gorgeous 6 foot 4, strapping 210, handsome young man, who walks and runs and plays and jumps around and holds hands with his girlfriend. And all of a sudden, you're going to take all of that away?"[27]

> **Some of the effects of the disease on the brain as well as other parts of the body may be subtle at first, not making themselves apparent for several years.**

Years of Disabilities

A 2001 study in Great Britain followed some 1,400 neonatal meningitis patients who survived the disease to see how it affected them later in life. The authors of the study learned that even years after recovering from the disease, many of the patients continued to show ill effects.

Meningitis is, after all, a disease that makes close contact with the brain. Some of the effects of the disease on the brain as well as other parts of the body may be subtle at first, not making themselves apparent for several years. Among the effects of meningitis that may not make themselves known for years, the study found, were hearing problems, behavioral issues, and strabismus, which is a visual defect that often results in the person becoming cross-eyed. "Although not as devastating as more disabling conditions, these are important problems that may adversely affect a child's well-being,"[28] wrote the authors of the study.

Many of the young children who survived meningitis turned out to be poor students. They suffered from learning disabilities: The study found that nearly 10 percent had difficulty learning language skills. Some of these students also suffered from hearing loss, which the authors of the study suggested may have a lot to do with why they were slow learners. Wrote the authors, "Children with speech and language problems also had hearing impairment, intellectual impairment, or both."[29]

The authors of the British study pointed out that there are no programs in Great Britain or most other countries that closely monitor young children after they recover from meningitis. The authors suggested that if a regular program of hearing tests can be established for them, their hearing problems may be discovered and corrected well before they fall behind in their studies.

Effects on Mental Health

Meningitis may result in more than just physical effects on its victims. Patients who spend weeks in isolation from others because of the contagious nature of the disease may fall into deep spells of depression. Depression is a mental illness characterized by feelings of sadness, hopelessness, and inadequacy. Depressed people may find themselves unable to get out of bed in the morning. They may want to hide in their own worlds, afraid to face others. Severely depressed people may contemplate or carry out suicidal acts. Or, they may lash out at others, voicing their frustration in anger and hostility.

British physician Trisha Macnair told the BBC, "It's very common to feel low after meningitis. There are several reasons for this: coming to terms with experiencing a traumatic event, accepting the possibility of permanent disabilities, the frustration of a slow recovery and simply the effect of the infection on the brain centers that control emotions. Anger, sadness, gloom, despondency, depression, anxiety—all these are quite common after meningitis."[30]

Therefore, in addition to undergoing treatment for the physical effects of meningitis many victims of the disease may also have to take antidepressant drugs or seek counseling from mental health experts, such as psychiatrists or psychologists. Their friends and family members may also find themselves helping the meningitis victims overcome their feelings of mental anguish.

> **Patients who spend weeks in isolation from others because of the contagious nature of the disease may fall into deep spells of depression.**

Indeed, as Oscar Wilde lay dying from meningitis, his longtime friend, Reginald Turner, didn't know quite what to make of the author's mental state. Turner often visited Wilde at his bedside. After one visit to the suffering author, Turner wrote a friend, "He has not once hinted he thinks he is in danger nor did he before the delirium began. He was only anxious to be out of pain. . . . He is very difficult and rude."[31]

Too Much for a Family to Bear

Sometimes, the effects of meningitis on the victim can overwhelm his or her family. Doctors, hospitals, and drugs are very expensive. Families without health insurance may find themselves facing tens of thousands of dollars in expenses. Even families with health insurance may also face stiff costs. For example, seven-year-old Waneshia Taylor lost both her legs to meningococcemia, which also left scars on her face and body. When the young girl from Waxahachie, Texas, arrived home from the hospital, her family members were hardly able to care for her in their modest home.

Waneshia's family was fortunate because their plight came to the attention of a local church. More than 100 volunteers from the Smith Chapel AME Church and other groups raised $70,000, then helped rebuild Waneshia's home, enlarging the house, modernizing its utilities, and adding wheelchair ramps, special bathroom fixtures, and other components that made the house handicap accessible. For example, the church members constructed an oversized shower stall. "It may seem a little large," project architect Don Murray told the *Dallas Morning News*, "but Waneshia's a child, and she'll need an adult to help her get around."[32]

> **Families without health insurance may find themselves facing tens of thousands of dollars in expenses. Even families with health insurance may also face stiff costs.**

With help from the community, Waneshia was able to settle into her new life. She has adjusted to life in a wheelchair, returning to school and learning to live with her disabilities. "Waneshia is fine," her mother, Wanda Johnson, told the *Dallas Morning News*. "She has a long way to go, but she's the one who keeps me going. She has never had a bad day since this happened."[33]

Widespread Panic

The example set by the church members in Waxahachie show that some communities respond positively to a meningitis case. In other communities, the reactions are quite different. It is not unusual for panic to spread throughout a community after a few cases of meningitis are reported.

In 1996 and 1997, Rhode Island experienced a higher than normal incidence of meningitis—a total of 47 cases were reported statewide, including 16 deaths. In early 1998, another 3 cases were reported, prompting state officials to organize a widespread vaccination program. Panic ensued, leading to long lines of people seeking vaccinations as well as anger when authorities ran short of the inoculations. Local politicians as well as health officials may have helped fuel the fear that soon spread across Rhode Island. They soon determined that none of the fatal cases were related—and that Rhode Island's meningitis rate was not that much higher than any other state in New England or the rest of the United States. However, health officials still believed a major epidemic could be brewing and announced a widespread plan to inoculate some 274,000 people—a quarter of the state's population—over a 6-month period.

> **When clinics ran out of the vaccine, emotions often turned ugly.**

Soon, people flocked to hospitals, clinics, and physicians' offices, where they waited in long lines for inoculations. When news reporters interviewed people waiting in line, they learned that few of them knew much about meningitis, its symptoms, or its consequences—but they all feared for their lives. When clinics ran out of the vaccine, emotions often turned ugly. Judith Peretti, the assistant administrator of one Rhode Island clinic, told NPR radio's *All Things Considered*, "We had one individual this morning kicking our door trying to get in, because she was so upset when we told her we didn't have any more vaccine. We have people calling up, calling us liars. There's a general panic."[34]

Meanwhile, people who intended to travel to Rhode Island canceled their plans out of fear they could contract the disease. Grandparents told their out-of-state grandchildren to stay away. In Rhode Island schools, teachers told children not to hold hands. During the panic, an editorial in Rhode Island's largest newspaper, the *Providence Journal*, admonished its readers, "We all need to calm down."[35] Eventually, the panic in Rhode Island did subside, and the vaccination program was carried out to its completion.

The Meningitis Belt

Even without the vaccine, the likelihood that meningitis would spread through entire American communities, infecting dozens or even hundreds of people, is remote. That is not the case in the African meningitis belt. Because of environmental conditions, the impoverished lifestyle found in large portions of Africa, the crowded housing, and the lack of health care available to many people in Africa, meningitis epidemics are a true cause for concern. Over the years, thousands of people have died in meningitis epidemics in sub-Saharan Africa.

> "Because of environmental conditions, the impoverished lifestyle found in large portions of Africa, the crowded housing, and the lack of health care available to many people in Africa, meningitis epidemics are a true cause for concern."

The World Health Organization has tracked trends in meningitis infections in Africa back to 1970, finding that epidemics in the belt last for some 3 or 4 years. Since then, major epidemics in the belt have broken out in 1977, 1986, and 1995, infecting hundreds of thousands of victims.

Such epidemics have had devastating consequences on the region. In addition to the loss of life, widespread epidemics of meningitis in the belt have broken up families, destroyed businesses and farms, added to the poverty of the region, and discouraged investment by foreign interests. One physician who worked as a volunteer for the humanitarian group Doctors Without Borders wrote about a sad case he found in one African village. He said, "We drove out of the compound early each morning to go and vaccinate in the villages. The little girl next door would wave till we disappeared round the corner. One morning she waved and grinned as usual, but by the time we got home in the evening she was near death."[36]

Overnight Epidemics

While the WHO's studies have indicated there is a pattern and something of a predictability to the meningitis epidemics in Africa, elsewhere outbreaks of the disease can occur virtually overnight. In such cases, a change in social conditions in a community is often at the root of the outbreak. For example, starting in the 1990s, Pacific Islanders emigrated to New Zealand—a country with little poverty, an adequate public health system, and little history of disease epidemics. The new immigrants came from the hundreds of islands scattered across the Pacific Ocean, including places such as Guam as well as the islands of Micronesia and Melanesia.

They arrived in New Zealand to find little housing available to them, and so in many cases large families were forced to share tiny homes. Often, a dozen or more people found themselves crowded into one-room apartments. That type of close contact led to several outbreaks of meningitis in the Pacific Islander population of New Zealand. The epidemic also afflicted the Maori, members of an ethnic group native to New Zealand. Dr. Diana Lennon, a pediatrician at the University of Auckland in New Zealand, told the PBS documentary *Nova*, "Although it's difficult to say cause and effect, it seems very likely that people crowded together have shared the infectious organism."[37]

Virtually overnight, emergency room doctors in New Zealand found themselves inundated with meningitis cases. Lennon told *Nova*, "A Pacific Island child born in Auckland has a one in a hundred chance of contracting meningococcal disease in his or her first year of life. And that's extraordinary."[38] In New Zealand, the infection rate continued to rise until 2003. Since 2003, the

> " Often, a dozen or more people found themselves crowded into one-room apartments. That type of close contact led to several outbreaks of meningitis in the Pacific Islander population of New Zealand. "

rate of infection has declined, thanks in large part to a widespread immunization program, but meningitis remains a major public health concern in New Zealand.

As Rhode Island's experience shows, meningitis is the type of disease that can cause widespread concern and even panic in many communities. In most cases, public health officials know how to contain the disease and ensure that it does not spread to others. In places like Africa and New Zealand, though, where vaccines and basic health care are often lacking, even the best efforts of physicians and health experts often fall short, leading to devastating consequences among the people afflicted with the disease.

Primary Source Quotes*

What Are the Social Impacts of Meningitis?

66 I remember going into John's room, and he was under. And I remember kissing him and saying, 'If you can't do this, if you can't make it through this, you go ahead and go. Mommy will understand. Don't stay for mommy, because I'll understand. But if you want to do this and you want to fight, we will fight this as a family.' 99

—Paige Kach, quoted in "Silent Killers," CBS News *48 Hours*, September 20, 2002.

Kach is the mother of Rhode Island college student John Kach, who lost a leg and a hand to meningococcemia.

66 The hardest thing was to walk to the cemetery, to see his name on a gravestone. His name shouldn't be on a gravestone. It should be on a wedding invitation, a birth announcement. 99

—Frankie Milley, quoted in Melissa Dahl, "Meningitis Threatens College Students," MSNBC.com, September 5, 2007. www.msnbc.com.

Milley is the mother of Ryan Milley, an 18-year-old Texas student who died of meningitis.

* Editor's Note: While the definition of a primary source can be narrowly or broadly defined, for the purposes of Compact Research, a primary source consists of: 1) results of original research presented by an organization or researcher; 2) eyewitness accounts of events, personal experience, or work experience; 3) first-person editorials offering pundits' opinions; 4) government officials presenting political plans and/or policies; 5) representatives of organizations presenting testimony or policy.

❝We initially went down and put in a hard day's work and thought we were going to make a difference. In the long term, we thought about what would make this child comfortable. It has become a labor of love.❞

—The Rev. James Ford, quoted in Sharon Egiebor, "A Gift for Waneshia: Church, Other Groups Do What It Takes to Help Girl Who Lost Her Legs," *Dallas Morning News*, April 21, 2001.

Ford's church raised $70,000 and spent 18 months renovating and expanding a home for 7-year-old meningococcemia victim Waneshia Taylor, who lost both legs to the disease.

❝You have to be a strong person, and you need quite a lot of support from others to get through it, because you think you've hit the end. You think you're never going to see the light at the end of the tunnel.❞

—Amy Mansell, quoted in *Nova*, "Killer Disease on Campus," September 3, 2002. www.pbs.org.

Mansell, 17, lost both legs and parts of both hands to meningococcemia.

❝It is essential that all cases of bacterial meningitis occurring during the first year of life are followed up fully so that children who require educational and other support are recognized at an early age.❞

—Dr. John de Louvois, quoted in Reuters Health Information, "Learning Disabilities Persist Among Teen Survivors of Infantile Meningitis," April 9, 2007. www.medscape.com.

De Louvois is co-author of a British study that assessed the mental and physical health of 1,400 survivors of neonatal meningitis.

"Most frequently hit are 18 countries in sub-Saharan Africa's so-called 'meningitis belt.' This is an area where the disease is endemic: meningitis is 'silently' present, and there are always a few cases."

—Doctors Without Borders, *International Activity Report 2001*, "Meningitis: Deadly Annual Epidemic in Africa's 'Meningitis Belt,'" 2001. www.doctorswithoutborders.org.

Doctors Without Borders is an international humanitarian organization that provides volunteer physicians to countries stricken by disease and warfare.

"Children are dying. Children are going through terrible illnesses. This is an incredibly significant epidemic for us."

—Dr. Wendy Walker, quoted in *Nova*, "Killer Disease on Campus," September 3, 2002, transcript accessed at www.pbs.org.

Walker is a physician at Middlemore Hospital in Auckland, New Zealand.

"It's almost a panic. People are very, very scared."

—Maxine White, quoted in Debbie Howlett, "Meningitis, Terror Strike in Ohio: 2 Teens Are Dead from the Bacteria, and Residents Are Approaching Panic," *USA Today*, June 5, 2001.

White's husband is pastor of an Alliance, Ohio, church, where half the congregation stayed home from services from fear that meningitis was spreading through the community.

66 Folks are very emotional because there is a large amount of fear out there. And I think the thing that amazes me is that they are not listening to the health professionals. 99

—Art Garnes, quoted in Linda Wertheimer, "Analysis: Thousands of Students and Teachers in Ohio Inoculated Against Bacterial Meningitis," *All Things Considered*, June 8, 2001.

Garnes, superintendent of schools in Alliance, Ohio, was criticized by parents for keeping schools open after two students died from meningitis.

66 Everybody's been kind of paranoid. It's just kind of getting frustrating because everything is rumors and nobody is getting any, like, solid information. 99

—Mary Ann Kibler, quoted in Linda Wertheimer, "Analysis: Thousands of Students and Teachers in Ohio Inoculated Against Bacterial Meningitis," *All Things Considered*, June 8, 2001.

Kibler is a student at Alliance High School in Ohio, where two of her classmates died of meningitis in 2001.

66 After a week in the hospital and ten days at home, I went back to school. No one else had been diagnosed with meningitis, but everyone I'd come in contact with in the two weeks before my ordeal—about 400 students—had to take antibiotics to ward off a potential infection. 99

—Sam Ellerbach, quoted in Beth Shapouri, "I Almost Died in My Dorm Room," *Cosmo Girl*, October 2007.

A student at Oklahoma State University, Ellerbach contracted meningitis in 2007.

66 There's the tremendous wind, which churns up a lot of dust, and then there is the heat. These are the conditions which make meningitis epidemics highly viable. **99**

—Jean Gabriel Wango, quoted in Brahima Ouedraogo, "Health-Africa: Meningitis Sweeping Through Burkina Faso," Global Information Network, August 3, 2002.

Wango is an official of the ministry of health of Burkina Faso, an African nation struck by a meningitis epidemic in 2002.

Facts and Illustrations

What Are the Social Impacts of Meningitis?

- The Indian capital of New Delhi experienced a meningitis panic in 2005 when **10 victims died** of the disease; thousands of people swarmed hospitals and clinics demanding immunizations.

- Between 1991 and 2007, more than **6,000 people**—mostly Pacific Islanders and members of the Maori ethnic group—have been afflicted with meningitis in New Zealand. Nearly 250 of those victims have died from the disease.

- A widespread panic in South Wales, a region of Great Britain, occurred in 1999 when **three deaths** from meningococcal disease were reported early in the year. Responding to public demands, the Welsh government initiated a comprehensive vaccination program.

- The massive meningitis immunization program initiated by Rhode Island cost state taxpayers some **$7 million**; about 274,000 people, most of them between the ages of 2 and 22, received vaccinations as part of the program.

- The Centers for Disease Control and Prevention regards an "outbreak" of a disease to consist of **10 cases per 100,000** people in a community.

- Many communities have initiated mass meningitis vaccination programs. These include Edmonton, Canada, which authorized vaccinations for anyone between the ages of **2 and 20** after 9 children died from meningitis in 1999 and 2000 and the Canadian province of Calgary, which **authorized vaccines** for all residents between the ages of 2 and 24 in 2001.

- In 2006, some **9,000** health care workers were assigned to vaccinate and treat people in Burkina Faso, where **19,000** people contracted meningitis, including **1,500** who died.

Was the 1998 Meningitis Panic in Rhode Island Justified?

The U.S. Centers for Disease Control and Prevention defines an outbreak of a disease to consist of at least 10 related cases in a population of 100,000 people. In 1996 and 1997, the rate of meningitis in Rhode Island was well below 3 cases per 100,000 people, and yet by early 1998, state officials had ordered a massive vaccination program. According to CDC statistics, other New England states experienced rates of meningitis that were slightly less than what occurred in Rhode Island. Those states did not order widespread inoculations.

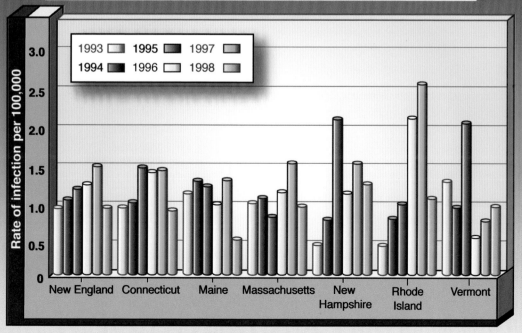

Source: U.S. Centers for Disease Control and Prevention, *Morbidity and Mortality Weekly Report*, "Meningococcal Disease–New England, 1993–1998," July 30, 1999. www.cdc.gov.

Pacific Islanders and Maori Most Afflicted Ethnic Groups in New Zealand

An epidemic of meningitis among the Pacific Islanders and Maori populations of New Zealand erupted in the 1990s, as many Pacific Islanders emigrated to Auckland and other cities, where they were forced to move into cramped housing. The epidemic hit a peak in 2001, when more than 500 cases were reported in New Zealand. By 2003, the effects of a vaccination program started showing results, and the number of cases began receding.

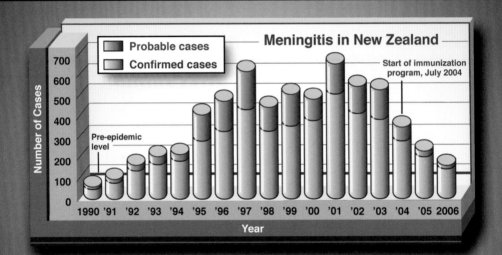

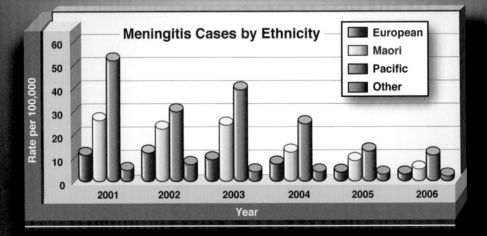

Source: Diana Martin, Liza Lopez, and Kerry Sexton, "The Epidemiology of Meningococcal Disease in New Zealand in 2006," New Zealand Ministry of Health, June 2007. www.moh.govt.nz.

- In 2004, to stem the epidemic of meningitis among Pacific Islanders and native Maori, the government of New Zealand initiated a national vaccination program that cost some **$200 million.**

- In Australia, government leaders were pressured by a public outcry to establish a meningitis vaccination program in 2002, which targeted a million young citizens for inoculations that cost about **$41 million.**

The Economic Cost of Meningitis

The U.S. Centers for Disease Control and Prevention released a study that attempted to place an economic cost on meningitis and treating its complications. For example, the study suggested that it costs society $200,000 to compensate for the amputation of an arm or leg. That cost stems from the fees charged by the doctor and hospital as well as the cost of rehabilitating the patient. A meningitis death costs $1.3 million—mostly from the loss of income the victim would earn in his or her lifetime.

	Total Costs of Acute Infection
Complication of Meningits	**Long-term costs**
Skin scarring	$40,288
Single amputation	$200,906
Multiple amputations	$453,860
Hearing loss	$344,889
Neurologic disability	$3,127,925
Death	$1,340,348
Average cost per person	**$34,590**

Source: Ismael Ortega-Sanchez, "The Economics of Adolescent Meningococcal Vaccination in the U.S.: Direct and Indirect Benefits," National Center for Immunization and Respiratory Diseases, June 2007. www.cdc.gov.

Long-Term Consequences of Neonatal Meningitis

A 2001 study by British researchers found that survivors of neonatal meningitis go on to experience a number of ill effects as they grow older, such as hearing problems; speech and language difficulties; and problems with their eyesight, such as strabismus, which is a visual defect that often results in the victim becoming cross-eyed. The study followed some 1,400 survivors of neonatal meningitis as they reached their teen years and beyond.

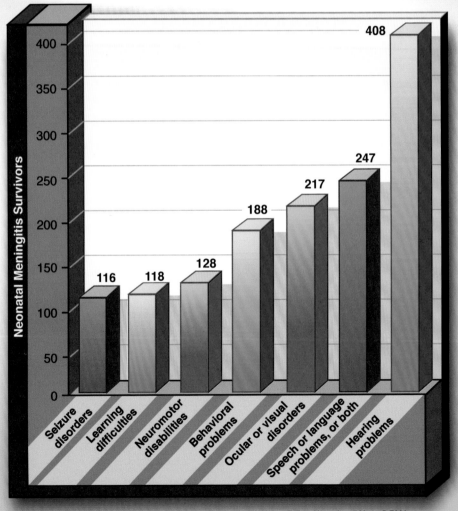

Source: Helen Bedford et al., "Meningitis in Infancy in England and Wales: Follow Up at Age 5 Years," *BMJ*, September 2001. www.pubmedcentral/nih.gov.

- During the meningitis panic that swept through Alliance, Ohio, in 2001, public health authorities administered **40,000 free doses** of antibiotic medications to frightened residents, *USA Today* reported.

- A study performed in Melbourne, Australia, found that **130 children** who survived meningitis achieved lower scores in school than children who had not been afflicted by the disease, the medical journal *BMJ* reported in 2001. The children were tested 7 and 12 years after their recoveries from meningitis.

- Moscow, Russia, suffered through a meningitis epidemic in 2003 when **251 people,** mostly children, contracted the disease; 22 cases were fatal. Authorities responded by ordering the vaccinations of **400,000 children** under the age of 8, the *Moscow Times* reported.

Can Meningitis Be Prevented?

Can Meningitis Be Prevented?

> **"** We're going to make a difference in this disease. It may take a few years to do it because it's very complex, but this is the right point in time with the right amount of science. **"**

—Dr. Brent Giroir, director of critical care, Children's Medical Center, Dallas, Texas.

Any college student who has made his or her way to the hospital emergency room, sick with fever, nauseous, and in pain from a splitting headache and very stiff neck, probably doesn't remember much about the early stages of treatment. Chances are, when the physician recognized the symptoms of meningitis, an intravenous drip of antibiotics was commenced immediately.

In the years since the discovery of penicillin, other antibiotic drugs have been developed. Penicillin is still widely used, but other drugs, such as ciprofloxacin and cefotaxime, have been found to be effective against meningitis. Ciprofloxacin works by breaking down the genetic material of the bacteria, thus rendering the germs harmless. Cefotaxime kills germs by interfering with the ability of the bacteria to form cell walls; without walls, the bacterial germs dissolve and die. Those drugs, as well as other antibiotics, can be used to fight meningitis and a number of bacterial infections.

The physician will decide the strength of the dosage for the meningitis patient, but most patients can expect to receive intravenous drips of antibiotic medication as many as four times a day. Depending on the severity of the infection, the treatments could last as long as three weeks.

Many antibiotic drugs have unpleasant side effects, including nausea, vomiting, and diarrhea. Some patients develop skin rashes, fever, and difficulty breathing from antibiotic drugs.

Whenever a case of meningitis surfaces, particularly on a college campus, health officials make attempts to find people who may have had close personal contact with the ill person. If they are located, those people are advised to take antibiotics in case they are already infected but not yet showing symptoms. Therefore, even people who don't show symptoms of meningitis—and may not, in fact, be infected—may have to endure unpleasant antibiotic drug treatments.

Meningitis is an unpleasant disease and the treatments for it can be unpleasant as well. However, if caught in time, meningitis can be treated with antibiotics with a high degree of success.

All Recruits Immunized

While meningitis can be successfully treated with antibiotics, if people are vaccinated against the disease they stand a very good chance of never being infected in the first place and forced to undergo unpleasant antibiotic treatments. The first vaccine for meningitis was administered on a wide scale in 1971. It was developed with the help of funding from the U.S. military. During the 1960s, new recruits were found to be highly susceptible to meningitis, mostly because of the close living conditions found in their barracks

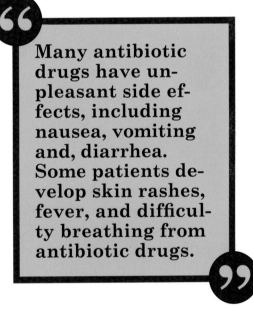

Many antibiotic drugs have unpleasant side effects, including nausea, vomiting and, diarrhea. Some patients develop skin rashes, fever, and difficulty breathing from antibiotic drugs.

during basic training. At the time, the infection rate among new inductees was 25 out of every 100,000 recruits. Starting in 1971, every inductee has been administered a meningitis vaccine and now, meningitis is virtually unknown in the U.S. military. Indeed, the infection rate among new recruits is now less than 1 per 100,000 inductees.

Several vaccines have been developed in recent years to prevent meningitis. Among the most common immunizations administered in the

United States are pneumococcal conjugate vaccine, or PCV7, and *Haemophilus influenzae* type b vaccine, or Hib, both of which may be given to children before they begin school; and pneumococcal polysaccharide vaccine, or PPV, which is given to teens and adults, and meningococcal conjugate vaccine, or MCV4, which is administered to teens who have not been previously vaccinated. In addition to meningitis, the Hib vaccine is effective against a number of other diseases caused by the Hib bacteria, including pneumonia as well as epiglottitis, which is a swelling of the tongue that could cause strangulation; cellulitis, which is a skin infection; pericarditis, an inflammation of the sac of fluid that surrounds the heart; empyema, a buildup of pus around the lungs; and osteomyelitis, a painful bone infection.

The discovery of the Hib vaccine in 1990 was a breakthrough, greatly reducing the spread of hemophilus meningitis and the other ailments. Development of the Hib vaccine commenced in the 1960s when two teams of researchers attacked the problem. One team was headed by David Smith, a Rochester, New York, physician specializing in infectious diseases, and Porter Anderson, a University of Rochester professor of bacteriology. The other team researching the vaccine was headed by John Robbins and Rachel Schneerson, who were based at the National Institutes of Health. By 1969, the two teams had each developed their own versions of the vaccine. Essentially, the vaccine stimulates the immune system of a young child by employing proteins to link another bacteria to the Hib bacteria. Proteins are the building blocks of all organisms. When the proteins link the new germs to Hib, the body is prompted to produce antibodies that protect the child from Hib.

> Even though the vaccine is believed to be just between 85 and 90 percent effective, it has greatly reduced the spread of hemophilus meningitis in the United States and other industrialized nations.

It took years of trials and refinements before the vaccine was ready for distribution. Development of the vaccine included a test on 100,000 infants and children in Finland in 1975. Other tests were performed in the 1980s. Finally, in 1990, the vaccine went into widespread use. Even though the vaccine is believed to be just between 85 and 90 percent effective, it has greatly reduced the spread of hemophilus meningitis in the United States and other industrialized nations. "The Hib vaccine work is a wonderful success story," Dr. Richard A. Insel, a pediatrics professor at the University of Rochester who worked closely with Smith and Anderson, told the *New York Times*. "I don't think people thought it would be this successful, almost eradicating the disease."[39]

> " Despite the constant media coverage of meningitis cases— and the occasional communitywide panic that ensues after cases are reported— mandatory vaccinations to guard schoolchildren against meningitis are not required by all states. "

Still Seeking Solutions

While the Hib vaccine has helped reduce the spread of hemophilus meningitis, medical science has not yet found solutions for eradicating other forms of the disease. There are vaccines available to protect against meningococcal meningitis; however, since the disease is rarely found in the United States, vaccinations are recommended only for people who travel to places where the incidence of the disease is high, such as the meningitis belt in Africa. Nevertheless, cases still occur in the United States. In 2007, a trade school student in West Chester, Pennsylvania, died after contracting meningococcal meningitis. Sadly, the student, Jeffrey Cox, had been immunized against other forms of meningitis. That was also the strain of meningitis that killed Anne Ryan, the University of Pennsylvania student. She had also received a meningitis vaccination prior to contracting the disease.

There are also vaccines available to treat pneumococcal meningitis, but they are not effective in children under the age of two. As for neonatal meningitis, which is contracted by infants shortly after their births, by 2007 no vaccine had been developed that would prevent infection by the Streptococcus group B bacteria, which causes most cases of neonatal meningitis.

Vaccinated for School

Despite the constant media coverage of meningitis cases—and the occasional communitywide panic that ensues after cases are reported—mandatory vaccinations to guard schoolchildren against meningitis are not required by all states. Indeed, 15 states as well as the District of Columbia do not require the Hib vaccinations or any other vaccinations for meningitis. Just 21 states require prospective college freshmen to obtain meningitis vaccinations or sign a waiver stating they understand the dangers of the disease if they do not receive inoculations. Eleven states—including some that do not require immunizations—require that schools provide parents with information about the disease and the benefits of immunization.

> "If a massive epidemic in the meningitis belt does occur, the WHO predicts its efforts to supply vaccinations to the region could fall short by more than 50 million doses."

Many American colleges have come to recognize the dangers that meningitis poses to students and, regardless of what local laws may require, insist that incoming freshmen and transfer students obtain meningitis immunizations before beginning classes. Said Dr. Phillip Barkley, director of student health at the University of Florida–Gainesville, "There's a vaccine that's available that can prevent 80 percent of the cases and we want college students, particularly those that are coming into college, to learn about this potentially devastating disease and the vaccine."[40]

If a freshman is unable to obtain an immunization from a family doctor before his or her first semester begins, the health centers at most American colleges will provide meningitis vaccines. Students without health insurance are often provided the shots free of charge. According to the American College Health Association, as many as 600,000 incoming freshmen receive meningitis vaccines each year.

Hib Initiative

People who live in the African meningitis belt as well as other developing nations must rely on others to provide supplies of the vaccine. The

World Health Organization often responds to crises, quickly providing vaccines to the belt when epidemics occur. Starting in 2006, the WHO commenced a 2-year campaign to supply 28 million doses of meningitis vaccine to people who live in sub-Saharan Africa. However, if a massive epidemic in the meningitis belt does occur, the WHO predicts its efforts to supply vaccinations to the region could fall short by more than 50 million doses.

Another group that is working to supply meningitis vaccinations to developing nations is the GAVI Alliance, formerly known as the Global Alliance for Vaccines and Immunizations. In 2005, GAVI launched the Hib Initiative, making low-cost Hib vaccines available to 72 developing nations in sub-Saharan Africa and elsewhere. The alliance is financed by several nations and private foundations, including the Bill and Melinda Gates Foundation, which was established by U.S. software billionaire Bill Gates and his wife.

The Hib Initiative quickly showed results. In 2006, the *Journal of the American Medical Association* published a study showing that widespread Hib immunizations in Kenya resulted in an 88 percent reduction in diseases caused by Hib infection, including meningitis. Karen Cowgill, a U.S. Centers for Disease Control and Prevention epidemic specialist and lead author of the study, said, "These results demonstrate the effectiveness of the Hib vaccine in reducing severe childhood illness and associated deaths in Kenya, and lead us to conclude that many more deaths could be averted in Africa if more countries added the vaccine to their routine immunization programs."[41]

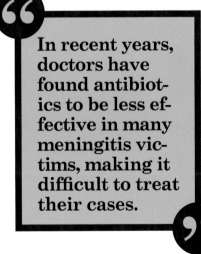

In recent years, doctors have found antibiotics to be less effective in many meningitis victims, making it difficult to treat their cases.

Research Continues

Meanwhile, research is continuing to find new ways to eradicate the disease. In Dallas, Texas, researchers have focused on the endotoxins released by the bacteria that cause meningitis. The endotoxins produced by the bacteria are chemicals that actually do the damage to the organs and other parts of the body. What makes meningitis such a horrific disease is that the amount of endotoxins released by the bacteria are as much as a thousand times greater than the endotoxins released by less-harmful bacteria, such as those that cause colds or flu.

At Children's Medical Center in Dallas, researchers have concentrated on blocking the release of endotoxins. They have found that increasing a natural protein found in white blood cells—which are natural infection fighters—can help block the release of endotoxins. The substance is known as bactericidal/permeability-increasing protein, or BPI. Dr. Brett Giroir, director of critical care at Children's Medical Center, told *Texas Monthly* magazine, "Antibiotics had always killed the bacterium itself effectively but they could do nothing about the toxins, which were prompting the fatal symptoms. The idea was to give the immune system some extra BPI to fight off this especially strong infection."[42]

In BPI therapy, the body's natural proteins would have to be artificially created and packed in massive doses into a medication. Research into BPI continues and is not likely to be approved for use for several years—if, indeed, it wins approval at all. The U.S. Food and Drug Administration studies new medications carefully and for very long periods. This is particularly true for medications administered to children, who would be the primary recipients of BPI drugs. Giroir believes BPI therapy holds great promise. It could mean that victims of meningococcemia may no longer face loss of limbs or other debilitating injuries. Also, young meningitis sufferers may be saved from the long-term consequences of the disease, such as hearing and eyesight loss and learning disabilities.

> " A student who goes to a lot of parties, gets little sleep, and puts off studying until the night before a big exam is not only risking a poor grade but is also very likely compromising his or her immune system. "

New Dangers

As medical researchers search for new methods to fight meningitis, they are also finding that some of the old methods are no longer guaranteed to be effective. People who have been administered antibiotics for other illnesses may have built up something of a resistance to them, making the drugs less effective the next time they are used. Bacteria is also known to evolve, making the germs resistant to antibiotic drugs. In recent years, doctors have found antibiotics to be less effective in many meningitis victims, making it difficult to treat their cases. Patients afflicted with pneumococcal meningitis have proven to be particularly difficult to treat. Dr. Moshe Arditi, a pediatrician at Cedars-Sinai Medical Center in Los Angeles and author of a study on drug-resistant bacteria, told *Science Daily,* "In the past several years in the United States, as well as worldwide, the pneumococcal (bacteria) that are resistant to antibiotics have been increasing in frequency—dramatically. Not only the frequency is increasing but the degree of resistance also is consistently becoming greater."[43]

To combat such drug-resistant germs, physicians often try administering several different antibiotics until they find one that works. In the meantime, science has been trying to keep up with the antibiotic-resistant germs. For example, the MCV4 vaccine is the newest immunization for meningitis; it has been in widespread use only since 2005.

Tips for Staying Germ-Free

The best way to avoid meningitis is for people to obtain the immunizations—particularly if they are teens preparing to leave for college. But prevention does not stop there—health officials agree that knowing the symptoms of meningitis can help victims obtain treatment before the disease has a chance to do much damage. Indeed, once students arrive at school, they may find themselves attending mandatory lectures led by the school's medical staff in which the symptoms of meningitis are explained.

Leading a healthy lifestyle also helps. Public health officials constantly counsel students and others to cover their mouths and noses when coughing or sneezing and to never drink from the same glasses or use the same eating utensils as other people. Also, health officials urge people to wash their hands often.

Finally, a student who goes to a lot of parties, gets little sleep, and puts off studying until the night before a big exam is not only risking a poor grade but is also very likely compromising his or her immune system. In such a harried and exhausted state, it wouldn't take much to contract a nasty case of cold or flu—or perhaps an infection that could be much worse, resulting in horrific consequences that can last a lifetime.

Can Meningitis Be Prevented?

❝How could a disease be so bad and kill so many children and adults, and leave children and adults maimed? How can it be so bad when we know that the bacteria that causes it is so susceptible to antibiotics?❞

—Dr. Brett Giroir, quoted in *Nova*, "Killer Disease on Campus," September 3, 2002, transcript accessed at www.pbs.org.

Giroir is director of critical care at Children's Medical Center in Dallas, Texas.

....

❝Our research shows that routine Hib vaccination is a feasible and highly effective way of preventing death related to Hib pneumonia and meningitis and could save the lives of a significant number of Asian children.❞

—Dr. Abdullah Baqui, quoted in GAVI Alliance news release, "Hib Vaccine: A Critical Ally in Asia's Effort to Reduce Child Deaths," June 28, 2007. www.gavialliance.org.

Baqui is associate professor at Johns Hopkins–Bloomberg School of Public Health in Baltimore, Maryland.

....

* Editor's Note: While the definition of a primary source can be narrowly or broadly defined, for the purposes of Compact Research, a primary source consists of: 1) results of original research presented by an organization or researcher; 2) eyewitness accounts of events, personal experience, or work experience; 3) first-person editorials offering pundits' opinions; 4) government officials presenting political plans and/or policies; 5) representatives of organizations presenting testimony or policy.

66We're talking very, very few people will be exempted from this.99

—Tom Kane, quoted in Shannon Colavecchio-Vansickler, "USF Tightens Vaccine Rules,"
St. Petersburg Times, November 28, 2007. www.sptimes.com.

Kane is director of residential services at the University of South Florida, which starting in 2008 made it mandatory for most students living on campus to be vaccinated against meningitis.

66Young people are exposed to many new experiences when they attend college, but meningitis should not be one of them.99

—Don White, quoted in "House Approves Bill to Prevent Meningitis on Campus,"
Pennsylvania State Senate news release, June 26, 2002. www.pasenategop.com.

White, a Pennsylvania state senator, is the author of the Pennsylvania law requiring students who live on campuses in that state to be vaccinated against meningitis.

66In developing countries where the incidence and mortality from bacteria meningitis far exceeds the rates in industrialized nations, the major barrier to immunization has been expense.99

—Allan R. Tunkel, *Bacterial Meningitis*. Philadelphia: Lippincott Williams & Wilkins, 2001.

Tunkel is a professor of internal medicine at Hahnemann University Hospital in Philadelphia and author of the book *Bacterial Meningitis*.

---

66 Maintain your immune system by getting enough rest, exercising regularly, and eating a healthy diet with plenty of fresh fruits, vegetables and whole grains.**99**

—Mayo Clinic, "Meningitis." www.mayoclinic.com.

The Mayo Clinic in Rochester, Minnesota, is one of the nation's premier medical treatment and research centers.

66 (The) World Health Organization is committed to eliminating meningococcal disease as a public health problem and ensuring control of sporadic cases through routine health services in the shortest possible time. The only way to reach this goal will be with an improved vaccine.**99**

—World Health Organization, "Fact Sheet: Meningococcal Meningitis," May 2003. www.who.int.

The World Health Organization is the public health arm of the United Nations.

66 If you are in contact with someone who has viral meningitis, the most effective method of prevention is to wash your hands thoroughly and often.**99**

—U.S. Centers for Disease Control and Prevention, "Viral ('Aseptic') Meningitis." www.cdc.gov.

The CDC is an agency of the U.S. government charged with monitoring threats to public health.

66We thought she'd be covered. They don't tell you that even if you get the vaccine, you're still susceptible.99

—Raymond Ortiz, quoted in Tania deLuzuriaga, "Despite Vaccine, Meningitis
Takes Teen's Life," *Boston Globe*, October 10, 2007.

Ortiz is the father of Bentley College freshman Erin Ortiz, who died from meningitis even though she had been vaccinated.

66The number of cases has increased in the last two years and we are likely to have major epidemics in a context of vaccine shortage.99

—Dr. Deo Nshimirimana, quoted in allAfrica.com, "Africa: WHO Predicts
Worst Meningitis Epidemic for Decade." http://allafrica.com.

Nshimirimana is director of communicable disease control for the World Health Organization in Africa.

66If this were a more minor illness, no, I couldn't justify it. But this is such a morbid disease, it causes such disruption. Every time there is a case, communities panic, it closes schools down.99

—Dr. Gregory Poland, quoted in "Feds Push New Meningitis Vaccine," CBS News, February 11, 2005. www.cbsnews.com.

Poland, a Minnesota physician, served on a U.S. Centers for Disease Control and Prevention panel that recommended all college freshmen living in dormitories be immunized against meningitis, despite the $100 per dose cost of the drug.

66When you choose not to get a vaccine, you're not just making a choice for yourself, you're making a choice for the person sitting next to you.99

—Dr. Lance Rodewald, quoted in Steve LeBlanc, "Parents Use Religion to Avoid Vaccines," Associated Press, October 18, 2007. http://news.yahoo.com.

Rodewald is director of the Immunization Services Division of the U.S. Centers for Disease Control and Prevention.

Can Meningitis Be Prevented?

- The Hib vaccine is believed to be **90 percent** effective in protecting people against hemophilus meningitis but because of limited availability in developing nations, the vaccine has reduced the rate of hemophilus meningitis by only **6 percent**.

- The only country in the world that vaccinates all its citizens against meningitis is Cuba. The Cuban government initiated the program in the 1980s. Since then, according to Cuban officials, **no children have died** from meningitis in the Caribbean country.

- As many as **40 percent** of the known strains of Streptococcus pneumonia, which are the bacteria that cause pneumococcal meningitis, are believed to be resistant to drugs.

- The largest mass meningitis immunization in history occurred in 1974 and 1975 when an epidemic in Brazil afflicted more than **250,000 people**, causing some **11,000** deaths. The government ordered vaccines administered to all **80 million** citizens of Brazil.

- In 2006, a manufacturing error resulted in the destruction of **20 million** doses of pneumococcal polysaccharide vaccine, also known as PPV, seriously hampering the ability of the World Health Organization to provide vaccinations to the African meningitis belt.

Which States Mandate Vaccinations for School Students?

A total of 15 states as well as the District of Colombia do not require public school students to obtain meningitis vaccinations. Meanwhile, 21 states require prospective college students to obtain the vaccinations before beginning classes or sign waivers stating that they understand the risk if they do not receive the vaccine. Connecticut, Indiana, and New Jersey require prospective college students to obtain the vaccinations, but permit students to turn down the treatments if they have religious or medical reasons that prevent them from receiving the inoculations. Fifteen states require schools, colleges, and summer camps to make information about the disease available to students and their parents.

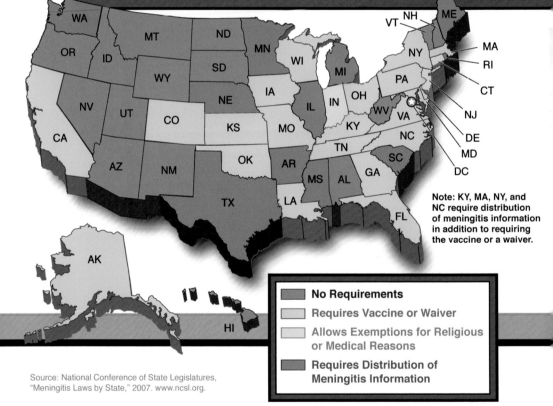

Note: KY, MA, NY, and NC require distribution of meningitis information in addition to requiring the vaccine or a waiver.

No Requirements

Requires Vaccine or Waiver

Allows Exemptions for Religious or Medical Reasons

Requires Distribution of Meningitis Information

Source: National Conference of State Legislatures, "Meningitis Laws by State," 2007. www.ncsl.org.

- A 2006 study by the U.S. Centers for Disease Control and Prevention reported that just **12 percent of teens** between the ages of 13 and 17 have received meningitis vaccines.

- The typical cost of the vaccine for meningitis is **$100**. About **600,000** college freshmen are immunized each year, which amounts to about **$60 million** a year to administer the meningitis vaccine just to college students.

- Many states allow parents to have vaccinations withheld from their children on religious grounds. In Massachusetts, **210 parents** requested religious exemptions for their children in 1996; in 2006, **474 parents** requested religious exemptions.

- Under state law in Virginia, college students who do not want to be vaccinated against meningitis can sign waivers turning down the inoculations; according to MSNBC, in 2001 **45 percent** of students signed waivers while in 2007, just **5 percent** signed waivers.

Antibiotic Treatment for Meningitis May Be Lengthy

Patients who contract meningitis may find themselves on antibiotic medications for as long as three weeks. Typically, the antibiotics are administered through an intravenous drip as many as four times a day. The drug therapy is often unpleasant: among the side effects are nausea, vomiting, diarrhea, skin rashes, fever, and difficulty breathing.

Microorganism causing meningitis	Duration of therapy
Streptococcus pneumoniae	10–14 days
Neisseria meningitidis	7 days
Streptococcus agalactiae	14–21 days
Listeria monocytogenes	21+ days
Haemohilus influenzae	7 days

Source: Allan R. Tunkel, *Bacterial Meningitis*. Philadelphia: Lippincott, Williams & Wilkins, 2001.

Four Common Meningitis Vaccines Administered in the United States

There are four common vaccines for meningitis administered in the United States. None are 100 percent effective, but public health officials believe that they can go a long way toward protecting most people from contracting meningococcal disease.

Haemophilus Influenzae Type B (Hib)

Required vaccine for all school-age children in 35 states. Usually, the vaccine is administered starting at two months of age. Helps prevent diseases caused by Hib bacteria, including meningitis, pneumonia, and several other illnesses.

Pneumococcal Conjugate (PCV7)

Many states require the vaccine for school-age children. Usually administered before the child reaches the age of 2 years. In addition, it is recommended for children between the ages of 2 and 5 who are susceptible to infections, including children who suffer from heart disease, lung disease, and cancer.

Pneumococcal Polysaccharide (PPV)

Administered to older children and adults, particularly adults over the age of 65. Younger adults and children who have weak immune systems are also urged to obtain the vaccine. Typically, young recipients of the PPV vaccine have suffered from heart disease, diabetes, sickle-cell anemia, or have had their spleens removed.

Meningococcal Conjugate (MCV4)

Recommended for young people between ages 11 and 18 who have not yet been vaccinated, including prospective college freshmen.

Source: Mayo Clinic, "Meningitis." www.mayoclinic.com.

- According to *U.S. News and World Report,* **87 percent** of American children between the ages of 19 and 35 months received meningitis vaccinations in 2006; in 2002, just **41 percent** of children in that age group were vaccinated.

Efficacy of Vaccines for Meningitis

Two major vaccines for meningitis were introduced in 1990 and 2005. Clearly, those vaccines have helped reduce the spread of meningitis in the United States as statistics from the U.S. Centers for Disease Control and Prevention indicate. In 1990, the first year the *Haemophilus influenzae* type B vaccine was made available, nearly 2,500 victims were infected with meningitis. After a brief rise in cases, due to more infections on college campuses, the rates of infection started declining. In 2005, the meningococcal conjugate vaccine was introduced. That year, just 1,245 victims contracted meningitis.

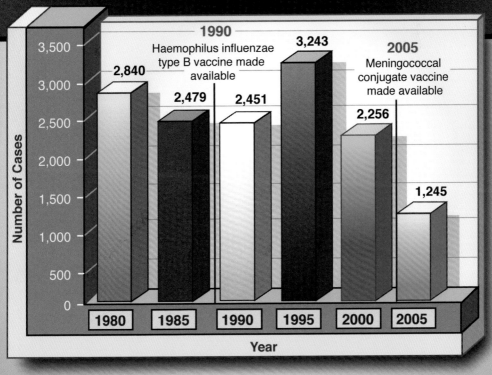

Source: U.S. Centers for Disease Control and Prevention, *Morbidity and Mortality Weekly Report,* "Summary of Notifiable Disease–United States, 2005," March 30, 2007. www.cdc.gov.

- About **30,000** hearing-impaired children who wear cochlcar implants were urged by the U.S. Food and Drug Administration in 2007 to obtain meningitis vaccinations; the electronic devices, which are implanted in the ears, can lead to infections that can cause meningitis.

- The pneumococcal conjugate vaccine was first administered in Great Britain in 2007; during the first year of the vaccine's use, British authorities believed they had saved at least **300 children** between the ages of two and four months from contracting meningitis, according to the BBC.

Key People and Advocacy Groups

American Academy of Pediatrics: The organization, which represents some 60,000 American pediatricians, encourages its members to support immunization programs. In addition, the organization provides its members with the latest information on trends in meningitis research and treatment. Also, the academy makes many resources about West Nile virus available to its members. West Nile virus, which is spread by mosquitoes, can lead to viral meningitis and encephalitis.

American College Health Association: The association, which represents some 900 colleges and universities in the United States, has emerged as the nation's chief advocacy group for vaccinating prospective college students and alerting them to the dangers of meningitis. Schools that belong to the association have committed themselves to making sure all incoming freshmen who expect to live in dormitories are vaccinated against meningitis.

Confederation of Meningitis Organizations (COMO): Based in Great Britain and Australia, the confederation was established in 2006 to develop a global strategy to eradicate meningitis. The confederation represents 20 meningitis advocacy groups based in 14 nations. COMO helps its member groups find resources to support meningitis education and provides them with the latest information about medical research and trends in the global meningitis fight.

Doctors Without Borders: The organization enlists physicians to provide emergency medical care in countries torn by war, famine, and natural disasters. The organization sends many teams of doctors each year into the African meningitis belt. One of the group's projects is to provide vaccination kits to doctors that ensure the drugs will be kept refrigerated. If the drugs are not kept refrigerated, they may spoil and have to be discarded. The kits outfitted by Doctors Without Borders include ice packs, coolers, generators, gas-powered refrigerators, freezers, and thermometers.

Alexander Fleming, Howard W. Florey, and Ernst Chaim: Alexander Fleming's discovery of penicillin in 1929 opened an important chapter in the understanding of how antibiotics fight infection. Oxford University physicians Howard W. Florey and Ernst Chaim refined Fleming's research, employing penicillin to kill germs. The three men shared the Nobel Prize for their work in fighting bacterial infections. Antibiotics have helped change meningitis from a disease that almost always meant death to one in which the mortality rate in industrialized nations is less than 10 percent.

Immunization Action Coalition: The coalition targets its programs at physicians and other health care professionals, encouraging them to expand their immunization efforts. The coalition publishes three journals—*Needle Tips, Vaccinate Adults,* and *Vaccinate Women*—that are circulated among 150,000 health care professionals, informing them of the latest developments in immunization science. Many of the articles in the coalition's publications include stories about survivors of meningitis as well as accounts by parents who lost sons and daughters to the disease.

Infectious Diseases Society of America: The society represents physicians, scientists, and others who work to control the spread of infectious diseases, including meningitis. The society publishes professional journals designed to keep its members abreast of the latest research in antibiotic medication and vaccines. The group is more than just a research society; the organization includes a lobbying arm, which works with lawmakers to increase government funding for infectious disease research and vaccination programs.

Helen Keller: Stricken by meningitis at the age of 19 months, Keller was left blind and deaf. She went on to become an author and activist for the rights of women, the handicapped, and others. Her story was dramatized in the Broadway play and Academy Award–winning film *The Miracle Worker.*

National Vaccine Information Center: Founded in 1982, the organization questions the effectiveness and safety of many vaccines and advocates placing the authority to approve vaccinations of children in the hands of parents. The group lobbied for passage of the National Vaccine Injury Act, which requires vaccine providers to furnish parents with written assessments of the benefits and risks of the vaccines and to ensure compensation to parents whose children are adversely affected by the immunizations.

David Smith, Porter Anderson, John Robbins, and Rachel Schneerson: Working independently, teams led by Smith and Anderson at a private research company in Rochester, New York, and by Robbins and Schneerson at the National Institutes of Health developed the vaccine that can fight diseases caused by the bacteria known as *Haemophilus influenzae* type b, or Hib. The Hib vaccine is less than 100 percent effective; nevertheless, it has helped to all but wipe out hemophilus meningitis in the United States and other industrialized nations.

Thomas Willis, Gaspard Vieusseux, and Anton Weichselbaum: The 3 doctors, working during eras in which medicine was based on little science, made important contributions to the understanding of meningitis. In 1661, Willis determined that meningitis was the cause of an epidemic that struck England and suggested the disease may be linked to cerebrospinal fluid. In 1805, Vieusseux reported the common symptoms of a meningococcemia epidemic that killed 33 people in Geneva, Switzerland. And in 1887, Weichselbaum, an Austrian, linked meningitis to a bacterial infection he cultured from a patient's cerebrospinal fluid.

Chronology

1887
Austrian Anton Weichselbaum links meningitis to a bacterial infection he cultures from a patient's cerebrospinal fluid.

About 2500 B.C.
Greek physician Hippocrates first notes the symptoms of meningitis in a patient and suggests the disease is linked to the lining of the brain.

1805
Swiss physician Gaspard Vieusseux reports the common symptoms of a meningococcemia epidemic that kills 33 people in Geneva.

1929
Alexander Fleming discovers penicillin; later Howard W. Florey and Ernst Chaim demonstrate penicillin's ability to kill germs.

1661
British physician Thomas Willis identifies the symptoms of meningitis in an epidemic and links the disease to cerebrospinal fluid.

1600   1700   1800   1900   1950

1882
Nineteen-month-old Helen Keller contracts meningitis and loses her hearing and eyesight; she will go on to become an author and activist.

1940–1945
Meningitis takes the lives of some 15,000 members of the military, making it the main cause of death among soldiers and sailors apart from battle.

1900
Author Oscar Wilde dies after suffering from meningitis for six weeks.

1559
French King Henry II dies of noncontagious meningitis after he sustains a head wound during a jousting competition; as he lingers near death, the king's doctors note their patient's painfully stiff neck, evidently unassociated with his wound.

1904 and 1905
Meningitis epidemic in New York City afflicts 6,700 victims, causing more than 5,000 deaths.

1971
The first vaccine for meningitis goes into widespread use as it is administered to U.S. military recruits; research of the vaccine had been financed by the military in response to a high rate of infection among inductees.

1969
Working independently, teams headed by David Smith and Porter Anderson at a Rochester, New York, company and by John Robbins and Rachel Schneerson at the National Institutes of Health develop the *Haemophilus influenzae* type b, or Hib, vaccine.

1998
After 3 young victims die of meningitis, Rhode Island officials react to public hysteria by ordering a statewide vaccination program for children; 274,000 young people are inoculated within 6 months.

1991
A long-lasting meningitis epidemic breaks out in New Zealand, afflicting more than 6,000 people, mostly Pacific Islanders and members of the Maori ethnic group; the infection rate starts declining in 2003.

2006
World Health Organization predicts sub-Saharan Africa is on the verge of a new meningitis epidemic.

1960   1970   1980   1990   2000

1974 and 1975
When an epidemic in Brazil afflicts more than 250,000 people, causing some 11,000 deaths, the government orders vaccines administered to all 80 million citizens of Brazil. It is the largest mass meningitis vaccination in history.

1990
Hib vaccine goes into widespread use, virtually eliminating hemophilus meningitis in the United States and other industrialized nations.

2005
Meningococcal conjugate vaccine, also known as MCV4, goes into widespread use in the United States; there are now four vaccines available to combat meningitis.

1977
The first of three major epidemics afflict the "meningitis belt" in sub-Saharan Africa; similar epidemics break out in 1986 and 1995, infecting as many as 250,000 victims.

2007
Some 22,000 people in Burkina Faso, a nation in West Africa, contract meningitis during the first 3 months of the year, including about 1,500 victims who die from the disease. A more widespread epidemic is avoided after the World Health Organization initiates an immunization program.

Related Organizations

Centers for Disease Control and Prevention (CDC)

Office of Communication

Building 16, D-42

1600 Clifton Road NE

Atlanta, GA 30333

phone: (800) 311-3435

e-mail: cdcinfo@cdc.gov

Web site: www.cdc.gov

The federal government's chief public health agency tracks infectious diseases in America. Numerous reports and studies on meningitis and related issues are available on the CDC's Web site.

Food and Drug Administration (FDA)

5600 Fishers Lane

Rockville, MD 20857-0001

phone: (888) 463-6332

Web site: www.fda.gov

The federal agency is charged with monitoring the safety of all drugs and medical tests performed in the United States. Visitors to the agency's Web site can learn about the FDA's assessments of new meningitis treatments, including the Xpert EV test, which will help doctors determine within hours whether a meningitis infection is viral or bacterial. In the past, doctors often had to wait a week or more to receive the results of a spinal tap.

GAVI Alliance

1130 Connecticut Avenue NW

Suite 1130

Washington, DC 20036

phone: (202) 478-1050

fax: (202) 478-1060

Web site: www.gavialliance.org

Formerly known as the Global Alliance for Vaccines and Immunization, GAVI Alliance is a consortium of international governments and private foundations that provide immunizations to people in developing nations. In 2005, GAVI launched the Hib Initiative, making low-cost Hib vaccines available to 72 developing nations in sub-Saharan Africa and elsewhere. Visitors to the organization's Web site can find reports on each country served by GAVI and learn how effective the group's work has been.

Meningitis Foundation of America

6610 Shadeland Station

Suite 200

Indianapolis, IN 46220

phone: (800) 668-1129

fax: (317) 595-6370

e-mail: support@musa.org

Web site: www.musa.org

The foundation raises money for meningitis research in the United States. Visitors to the Web site can find updates on meningitis research as well as links to other groups that support meningitis research in the United States and other countries.

Meningitis Research Foundation

Midland Way

Thornbury

Bristol

United Kingdom

BS35 2BS

phone: 01 45 428 1811

fax: 01 45 428 1094

e-mail: info@meningitis.org

Web site: www.meningitis.org

Great Britain has an aggressive program aimed toward vaccinations and early identification of meningitis patients. The foundation supports medical research in Great Britain and elsewhere. Visitors to the Web site can find many resources about the disease, including an explanation of symptoms, identification of people most at risk, causes of the disease, and how it is treated and prevented. Survivors of the disease have also posted their personal stories on the Web site.

National Center for Health Statistics

3311 Toledo Road

Hyattsville, MD 20782

phone: (800) 232-4636

e-mail: nchsquery@cdc.gov

Web site: www.cdc.gov/nchs

Part of the CDC, the center compiles statistics and reports on meningitis and many other diseases and health-related topics. The report *Health, United States 2006*, which includes statistics on diseases common in the United States, including meningitis, can be downloaded from the center's Web site.

National Foundation for Infectious Diseases

4733 Bethesda Avenue

Suite 750

Bethesda, MD 20814

phone: (301) 656-0003

fax: (301) 907-0878

e-mail: info@nfid.org

Web site: www.nfid.org

Founded in 1973, the organization works to educate the public and medical professionals about the latest trends in infectious diseases. By entering *meningitis* in the Web site's search engine, and then following the link for "Consumer Resources," visitors can find many reports, articles, and other resources about meningitis, including a National Public Radio interview with Dr. Jeanne Santoli, an immunization specialist for the U.S. Centers for Disease Control and Prevention, explaining the importance of meningitis vaccinations.

National Institutes of Health

9000 Rockville Pike

Bethesda, MD 20892

phone: (301) 496-4000

e-mail: NIHinfo@od.nih.gov

Web site: www.nih.gov

The National Institutes of Health is the chief funding arm of the federal government for medical research. Many resources about meningitis are available on the agency's Web site by accessing the Meningitis and Encephalitis Information Page, where visitors will find brief explanations of the diseases, information on how they are treated, and updates on new research into controlling the bacterial and viral infections that cause the two diseases.

National Meningitis Association (NMA)

738 Robinson Farms Drive

Marietta, GA 30068

phone: (866) 366-3662

fax: (877) 703-6096

e-mail: support@nmaus.org

Web site: www.nmaus.org

The organization was founded by five mothers whose teenage children either died or lost limbs to meningococcal disease. The group is dedicated to spreading information about the dangers of meningitis and the importance of obtaining vaccines. By accessing the "Meningitis Aware-ness State by State" link, visitors to the group's Web site can learn about immunization laws in their state as well as find contact information for local NMA leaders.

World Health Organization (WHO)

Avenue Appia 20

CH - 1211 Geneva 27

Switzerland

phone: 41 22 791 2111

fax: 41 22 791 3111

e-mail: info@who.int

Web site: www.who.int

WHO is the public health arm of the United Nations. The agency tracks the spread of diseases across the globe and responds to many public health crises, such as rushing vaccines to impoverished or war-torn nations during epidemics. Visitors to the organization's Web site can download reports and updates about the ongoing efforts to eradicate meningitis in sub-Saharan Africa and elsewhere.

For Further Research

Books

Dan Bartolotti, *Hope in Hell: Inside the World of Doctors Without Borders.* Richmond Hill, Ontario: Firefly Books, 2006.

Barbara Belford, *Oscar Wilde: A Certain Genius.* New York: Random House, 2000.

Kevin Brown, *Penicillin Man: Alexander Fleming and the Antibiotic Revolution.* Gloucestershire, England: Sutton Publishing, 2005.

Margaret C. Fisher, editor, *Immunizations & Infectious Diseases.* Elk Grove Village, IL: American Academy of Pediatrics, 2006.

Matthias Frosch and Martin C.J. Maiden, editors, *Handbook of Meningococcal Disease.* Weinheim, Germany: Wiley-VCH, 2006.

Helen Keller, *The Story of My Life.* New York: Bantam Books, 1990.

James N. Parker and Philip M. Parker, editors, *The Official Patient's Sourcebook on Meningitis.* San Diego: ICON Health Publications, 2002.

Allan R. Tunkel, *Bacterial Meningitis.* Philadelphia: Lippincott Williams & Wilkins, 2001.

Carol Turkington, *The Brain and Brain Disorders.* New York: Facts On File, 2002.

Carol Turkington and Bonnie Lee Ashby, *The A to Z of Infectious Diseases.* New York: Checkmark Books, 2007.

Periodicals

The Australian, "Vaccines for a Million Children: $41 Million War Against Meningococcal Disease," August 20, 2002.

Helen Bedford et al., "Meningitis in Infancy in England and Wales: Follow Up at Age 5 Years," *BMJ*, September 2001.

BMJ, "Legacy of Bacterial Meningitis in Infancy: Many Children Continue to Suffer Functionally Important Deficits, " September 2001.

David Bruce, "Meningitis: Student Scourge Can Kill If Not Treated Promptly," *Erie Times News*, September 10, 2007.

Tania de Luzuriaga, "Despite Vaccine, Meningitis Takes Teen's Life," *Boston Globe*, October 10, 2007.

Kathleen Doheny, "It's Not Too Late in the Year for the Meningitis Vaccine," *Baxter (Arkansas) Bulletin*, October 2, 2007.

Julie Weingarden Dubin, "It Could Happen to You: 'I Almost Died from Dorm Disease,'" *Cosmopolitan*, April 2007.

Colleen Dunn and John Sullivan, "Meningitis Victim Etched in Memory," *Philadelphia Inquirer*, September 11, 2007.

Sharon Egiebor, "A Gift for Waneshia: Church, Other Groups Do What It Takes to Help Girl Who Lost Her Legs," *Dallas Morning News*, April 21, 2001.

C. Eugene Emery Jr., "As Schools Reopen, Students Warned: Wash Your Hands," *Providence Journal*, January 8, 2007.

Carolyn Gard, "What Is Meningitis?" *Current Health 2*, April/May 2003.

Debbie Howlett, "Meningitis, Terror Strike in Ohio: 2 Teens Are Dead from the Bacteria, and Residents Are Approaching Panic," *USA Today*, June 5, 2001.

Rebecca Kaplan, "Health Alerts Accompany Tribute: Overview of Meningitis Shows Disease Most Common Among College Students," *Daily Pennsylvanian*, September 11, 2007.

Perri Klass, "To Worry or Not?" *Parenting*, November 2002.

Brobson Lutz, "Meningitis: A Bacterial Killer," *New Orleans Magazine*, July 2003.

Donna A. MacMillan et al., "Community-Acquired Bacterial Meningitis in Adults: Categorization and Timing of Death," *Clinical Infectious Diseases*, October 2002.

Hannah McCouch, "I Almost Died of Dorm Disease," *Cosmopolitan*, April 2002.

Katherine Partridge, "The Meningitis Menace: It's a Frightening Illness That Can Be Both Swift and Deadly. The Good News Is There Are Ways to Protect Your Kids," *Today's Parent*, August 2002.

Cheryl Powell and Dave Ghose, "About 37,000 Ohioans Line Up for Drugs to Prevent Meningitis," *Akron Beacon Journal*, June 4, 2001.

Beth Shapouri, "I Almost Died in My Dorm," *Cosmo Girl*, October 2007.

Judith Woods, "The Menace of Meningitis," *London Telegraph*, March 9, 2007.

Internet Sources

American College Health Association, "Meningitis on Campus," April 27, 2005. www.acha.org/projects_programs/meningitis/studentnews2.cfm.

BBC, "The Meningitis Files," January 31, 2000. http://news.bbc.co.uk/2/hi/health/293298.stm.

International Activity Report 2001, "Meningitis: Deadly Annual Epidemic in Africa's 'Meningitis Belt,'" Doctors Without Borders, 2001. http://doctorswithoutborders.org/publications/ar/i2001/meningitis.cfm.

Nova, "Killer Disease on Campus," September 3, 2002. www.pbs.org/wgbh/nova/meningitis.

Jennifer Steinberg, "Stories of Discovery: Hib Vaccine," National Institutes of Health Office of Science Education. http://science.education.nih.gov/home2.nsf/Educational+ResourcesResource+FormatsOnline+Resources+High+School/BEB8326ABA992481852570F30071D67A.

Source Notes

Overview

1. Quoted in Judith Woods, "The Menace of Meningitis," *London Telegraph*, March 9, 2007. www.telegraph.co.uk.
2. Quoted in American College Health Association, "Meningitis on Campus," April 27, 2005. www.acha.org.
3. Brian R. Plaisier et al., "Post-Traumatic Meningitis: Risk Factors, Clinical Factors, Bacteriology, and Outcome," *Internet Journal of Neurosurgery*, 2005. www.ispub.com.
4. *World Health Organization Weekly Epidemiological Record*, "Risk of Epidemic Meningitis in Africa: A Cause for Concern," March 9, 2007, p. 79.
5. Quoted in Carolyn Gard, "What Is Meningitis?" *Current Health 2*, April/May 2003, p. 28.
6. Quoted in *Nova*, "Killer Disease on Campus," September 3, 2002, transcript accessed at www.pbs.org.
7. Helen Bedford et al., "Meningitis in Infancy in England and Wales: Follow Up at Age 5 Years," *BMJ*, September 2001, p. 3.
8. Quoted in Reuters Health Information, "Learning Disabilities Persist Among Teen Survivors of Infantile Meningitis." www.medscape.com.
9. Quoted in Nikki Roberti, "Health Services Offer Meningitis Vaccinations," *The Appalachian*, Sept. 20, 2007. http://theappstate.edu.
10. Quoted in American College Health Association, "Meningitis on Campus." www.acha.org.

How Does Meningitis Affect People?

11. Quoted in Hannah McCouch, "I Almost Died of Dorm Disease," *Cosmopolitan*, April 2002, p. 156.
12. Quoted in McCouch, "I Almost Died of Dorm Disease," p. 156.
13. Quoted in Colleen Dunn and John Sullivan, "Meningitis Victim Etched in Memory," *Philadelphia Inquirer*, September 11, 2007, B-2.
14. Quoted in Dunn and Sullivan, "Meningitis Victim Etched in Memory," B-1.
15. Quoted in Marie McCullough, "Penn Student's Diagnosis 'Was Wrong,' Says Lawyer," *Philadelphia Inquirer*, October 2, 2007, B-1.

How Prevalent Is Meningitis?

16. Quoted in Allan R. Tunkel, *Bacterial Meningitis*. Philadelphia: Lippincott Williams & Wilkins, 2001, p. 6.
17. Quoted in Tunkel, *Bacterial Meningitis*, p. 5.
18. Helen Keller, *The Story of My Life*. New York: Bantam Books, 1990, p. 4.
19. Keller, *The Story of My Life*, p. 4.
20. World Health Organization, "Fact Sheet: Meningococcal Meningitis," May 2003. www.who.int.
21. World Health Organization, "Fact Sheet: Meningococcal Meningitis," may 2003. www.who.int.
22. Quoted in David Bruce, "Meningitis: Student Scourge Can Kill If Not Treated Promptly," *Erie Times News*, September 10, 2007, p. 1.

23. Quoted in Gard, "What Is Meningitis?" p. 28.

24. Quoted in BBC News, "Hajj Meningitis Cases Fall," January 13, 2003. http://news.bbc.co.uk.

What Are the Social Impacts of Meningitis?

25. Quoted in "Silent Killers," CBS News *48 Hours*, September 20, 2002.

26. Quoted in "Silent Killers."

27. Quoted in "Silent Killers."

28. Bedford et al., "Meningitis in Infancy in England and Wales: Follow Up at Age 5 Years."

29. Bedford et al., "Meningitis in Infancy in England and Wales: Follow Up at Age 5 Years."

30. Quoted in "Doctor's Advice: Recovery from Meningitis," *BBC Health*, January 2007. www.bbc.co.uk.

31. Quoted in Barbara Belford, *Oscar Wilde: A Certain Genius.* New York: Random House, 2000, p. 303.

32. Quoted in Sharon Egiebor, "A Gift for Waneshia: Church, Other Groups Do What It Takes to Help Girl Who Lost Her Legs," *Dallas Morning News*, August 21, 2001.

33. Quoted in Egiebor, "A Gift for Waneshia: Church, Other Groups Do What It Takes to Help Girl Who Lost Her Legs."

34. Quoted in NPR *All Things Considered*, "Rhode Island Meningitis Panic," February 27, 1998, A-10.

35. Quoted in Tom Verde, "Alarmed by Meningitis, Rhode Island Tries Mass Inoculation," *New York Times*, March 8, 1998, A-10.

36. Quoted in Doctors Without Borders, *International Activity Report 2001*, "Meningitis: Deadly Annual Epidemic in Africa's 'Meningitis Belt,'" 2001. www.doctorswithoutborders.org.

37. Quoted in *Nova*, "Killer Disease on Campus." www.pbs.org.

38. Quoted in *Nova*, "Killer Disease on Campus." www.pbs.org.

Can Meningitis Be Prevented?

39. Quoted in Karen Freeman, "David H. Smith, 67, Developer of Vaccine Against Meningitis," *New York Times*, March 1, 1999, A-19.

40. Quoted in American College Health Association, "Meningitis on Campus." www.acha.org.

41. Quoted in GAVI Alliance news release, "Routine Use of Hib Vaccine Could Lead to Virtual Elimination of Killer Disease in Africa," August 9, 2006. www.gavialliance.org.

42. Quoted in Jim Atkinson, "Bad Blood," *Texas Monthly*, April 1999, p. 60.

43. Quoted in *Science Daily*, "Bacteria Becoming Increasingly Resistant to Antibiotics, but New Vaccines Are on the Horizon," January 14, 1999.

List of Illustrations

Index

Index

About the Author

Hal Marcovitz, a writer based in Chalfont, Pennsylvania, has written more than 100 books for young readers. His other titles in the Compact Research series include *Hepatitis* and *Phobias.*